Against Health

BIOPOLITICS

Medicine, Technoscience, and Health in the 21st Century

General Editors: Monica J. Casper and Lisa Jean Moore

Missing Bodies: The Politics of Invisibility
Monica J. Casper and Lisa Jean Moore

Against Health: How Health Became the New Morality
Jonathan M. Metzl and Anna Kirkland, Editors

Against Health

How Health Became the New Morality

Jonathan M. Metzl and Anna Kirkland

EDITORS

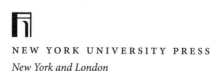

NEW YORK UNIVERSITY PRESS
New York and London

NEW YORK UNIVERSITY PRESS
New York and London
www.nyupress.org

References to Internet websites (URLs) were accurate at the time of writing.
Neither the author nor New York University Press is responsible for URLs
that may have expired or changed since the manuscript was prepared.

Library of Congress Cataloging-in-Publication Data

Against health : how health became the new morality /
edited by Jonathan M. Metzl and Anna Kirkland.
p. cm. — (Biopolitics, medicine, technoscience, and health in the 21st century)
Includes bibliographical references and index.
ISBN 978-0-8147-9592-7 (cl : alk. paper)
ISBN 978-0-8147-9593-4 (pb : alk. paper)
ISBN 978-0-8147-6110-6 (e-book : alk. paper)
1. Health—Moral and ethical aspects. 2. Medical ethics.
3. Health services accessibility. 4. Social medicine.
I. Metzl, Jonathan, 1964– II. Kirkland, Anna Rutherford.
RA418.A53   2010
362.1—dc22   2010018812

New York University Press books are printed on acid-free paper,
and their binding materials are chosen for strength and durability.
We strive to use environmentally responsible suppliers and materials
to the greatest extent possible in publishing our books.

Manufactured in the United States of America
c   10 9 8 7 6 5 4 3 2 1
p   10 9 8 7 6 5 4 3

To Carol Boyd, with deep gratitude

Contents

Acknowledgments

Against Health was a concept, and a conference, before it was a book. The editors express tremendous gratitude to the many people whose dedication, skill, generosity, and foresight enabled this transformation. From the beginning, Carol Boyd and David Halperin envisioned and supported the Against Health conference, which took place in October 2006 at the University of Michigan. Colleagues including Wendy Bostwick, Anne Esacove, Sasha Feirstein, Sean McCabe, Michele Morales, Justin Schmant, Lisa Kane Low, and Michelle McClellan served on the conference planning committee. In addition to the authors in this volume, Paul Campos, John Carson, Kenneth Warner, Susan Kippax, Paula Allen-Mears, Joycelyn Elders, Roddey Reid, Rebecca Herzig, Libby Bogdan-Lovis, Ray De Vries, Petra Kuppers, Magdalena Harris, Bernice Hausman, Michele Morales, Moya Bailey, Nicholas King, Brad Lewis, Lisa Kane Low, Susan Love, Elizabeth Roberts, and Kane Race contributed to the conference conversation in brilliant and challenging ways. Sacha Feirstein and Terri Torkko coordinated the whole event through the offices of the Univrsity of Michigan's Institute for Research on Women and Gender. At NYU Press, editor Ilene Kalish, and editorial assistant Aiden Amos, served as amazing advocates. And, perhaps most important, our remarkable and extraordinary graduate student assistant, Burke Hilsabeck, pulled the chapters into final coherence and, ultimately, pulled us through. Thank you all.

Introduction

Why Against Health?

JONATHAN M. METZL

How can anyone take a stand against health? What could be wrong with health? Shouldn't we be *for* health?

On behalf of the authors, let me reply to these questions by proclaiming that we believe that anyone who feels ill before, during, or after reading this book should seek immediate medical attention. We believe in the germ theory of infectious illness. We believe in penicillin. We believe that physicians should wash their hands between patient visits. We are optimistic about the promise of stem cell research. We believe that the transition from the rigid sigmoidoscope to the lower abdominal MRI represents indisputable progress. We are for bike helmets, sunscreen, and enteric-coated tablets, and we are against the swine flu. Perhaps most of all, we believe that disparities in incidence and prevalence of disease are closely linked to disparities in income and social support. We believe that documents such as the Department of Health and Human Services' "Healthy People 2010" prove beyond doubt that access to health care and availability of adequate health insurance remain unattainable goals for many Americans. We believe that such disparities need to be rectified, and we stand firmly behind recent expansions in healthcare coverage.

At the same time, we believe that defining the mission of this book solely as a call for redistribution of healthcare resources is to miss part of the point. That is because arguments supporting the reallocation of resources understandably assume that health is a fixed entity that can be transported from one setting to another. The rich have health, for instance, and the poor do not. While valid, such claims overlook the ways in which *health* itself is part of the problem that we mean to address.

As recent political debates in the United States have demonstrated, "health" is a term replete with value judgments, hierarchies, and blind assumptions that speak as much about power and privilege as they do about well-being. Health is a desired state, but it is also a prescribed state and an ideological position. We realize this dichotomy every time we see someone smoking a cigarette and reflexively say, "smoking is bad for your health," when what we really mean is, "you are a bad person because you smoke." Or when we encounter someone whose body size we deem excessive and reflexively say, "obesity is bad for your health," when what we mean is not that this person might have some medical problem, but that they are lazy or weak of will. Or when we attend town-hall meetings or Tea Party mosh pits and reflexively shout down other people for not understanding health care, when what we mean is that these people must be principally or politically misguided. Or even when we see a woman bottle-feeding an infant and reflexively say, "breastfeeding is better for that child's health," when what we mean is that the woman must be a bad parent. In these and other instances, appealing to health allows for a set of moral assumptions that are allowed to fly stealthily under the radar. And the definition of our own health depends in part on our value judgments about others. We see them—the smokers, the overeaters, the activists, and the bottle-feeders—and realize our own health in the process.

I have developed a strategy to help answer the question, *why against health*? When I am posed this question by friends, relatives, or even patients, I reply by asking my interlocutors to, for one day, pay attention to the *uses* of health in their daily lives. Where does the term appear? I ask. To what means and to what ends? This brief exercise is meant to complicate assumptions about health as a transparent, universal good. Instead, even the most cursory examination of health in daily conversation, email solicitation, or media representation demonstrates how the term is used to make moral judgments, convey prejudice, sell products, or even to exclude whole groups of persons from health care.

For instance, if after reading this book you walk to the nearest newsstand in search of health-themed magazines, you will undoubtedly find such popular periodicals as *Health*, *Healthy Living*, or *Men's* and *Women's Health*. It will not take much browsing time to realize that these publications share the common assumption that health is intimately connected to, and ultimately defined by, a person's appearance. These and other magazines commonly promote the message that healthy appearances embody a set of norms that are at once wholly mainstream and impossible to attain.

A recent issue of *Health* asks readers to consider whether, in the name of "beauty," they would consider having plastic surgery on their toes, or whether they would consider getting facials on their "fannies" to reduce cellulite. The magazine opines on such topics as "the best jeans for your body," "secrets to a good hair day," and "in search of the perfect bra," while inviting readers to share their weight-loss stories by divulging secret tips and by submitting before and after photographs that illustrate how their health has changed since their weight loss. *Men's Health* meanwhile subdivides health into the categories of Sex, Fitness, and Nutrition and instructs readers on ways to obtain buns of steel or build "razor sharp abs" in an effort to "get noticed," and then get laid, by the girl next door.[1]

Calling such language *sexism* or *cultural narcissism* would mobilize a particular critique. But calling it *health* allows these and other magazines to seamlessly construct certain bodies as desirable while relegating others as obscene. The result explicitly justifies particular corporeal types and practices, while implicitly suggesting that those who do not play along suffer from ill health. The fat, the flaccid, and the forlorn are unhealthy, the logic goes, not because of illness or disease, but because they refuse to wear, fetishize, or aspire to the glossy trappings of the health of others.

You might also log on to your computer only to be accosted by spam emails or pop-up Websites advertising a wide variety of tumescents that promise "sexual health." You might learn that information about erectile dysfunction (ED) "can be an important first step toward better sexual health," and that the second step involves ingestion of prescription Cialis™: "With CIALIS you can have the option of being ready fast . . . or have up to 36 hours to relax and take your time."[2] Or you might be directed to the Website of the "non-prescription all natural supplement" Ezerex, which promises a "rock-hard erection" in just twenty-five minutes: "EZEREX is made to act FAST like a prescription, but without all the unhealthy side effects!" The site further explains that the supplement "should be taken as part of a healthy lifestyle" and offers testimonials from men such as "David W.," who exclaims, "I don't have an ED problem but I do have a girlfriend who is 20 years younger than I am and she has an endless appetite for sex. I needed an edge and some extra help to keep up. EZEREX is her new best friend! Thank you."[3]

Calling such claims *phallocentrism* might mobilize a particular critique. But calling them *health* allows the Websites to construct social physiologies in which health is marked by the ability to stand at osseous attention for seemingly unhealthy periods of time, while unsubtly suggesting that the inability to do so indicates some sort of disease.

A different notion of health appears when you turn on your television and see public health advertisements that implore you to stop smoking by appealing to the health of your children. One recent Michigan campaign shows children left alone in homes or in cars, where they are helplessly left to breathe the second-hand smoke of their parents. The children speak dejectedly into the camera about the impact of their passively attained nicotine habits. "I smoke while I'm watching cartoons," says one girl in front of a television. "We smoke on the way to school," add two sisters trapped in a car. "When you smoke around your kids," the narrator explains, "it's like they're smoking."[4]

Calling such appeals *moralism* might mobilize a particular critique, and to be sure, the ads importantly confront the pernicious effects of second-hand smoke. But calling them *health* allows these campaigns to make a much wider set of assumptions about people who smoke as being irresponsible or negligent parents, parents who leave their children alone in cars or slowly kill them via their own solipsistic addictions. Pleural health is closely aligned with decency in this formulation, while the disease of smoking decays the body as well as the soul.

Finally, you might be sitting in an airport where, in lieu of an explanation for your flight delay, you are handed a complimentary copy of the *Wall Street Journal*, which contains the front-page headline, "Lighten Up: Pepsi Sales Force Tries to Push 'Healthier' Snacks in Inner City." According to the article, sales representatives for PepsiCo, Incorporated began a multimillion-dollar campaign to promote Baked Cheetos, Doritos, and Ruffles in the "inner city." "32% of adult Americans are obese," the article reads, and in response, PepsiCo hopes to encourage "inner-city African Americans and Latinos" to forgo the 25-cent packs of Flamin' Hot Cheetos and Nacho Cheese Doritos known fondly as "quarters," and to instead select lower-fat (and higher cost) offerings produced by the same company.[5]

Calling this approach *racism* or *capitalism* or any number of other -*isms* would mobilize a particular critique. But calling it *health* allows for a language of betterment that skillfully glosses over the structural violence done to minority and lower-income Americans, while at the same time suggesting that social and economic misfortune results from poor food choices. Calling it health also enables troubling slippages between the health of individual bodies and the health of economic ones, inasmuch as consumption of the very foods that (dubiously) help minority populations slim down also produce portly profits for PepsiCo Incorporated.[6]

The aim of this book might be divided into two parts, the first of which is exponentially easier than the second. First, we mean to unpack health and to explore the ideologies, structures, base pairs, and blind assumptions involved in its construction. Numerous theoretical tools hang at the ready in this regard. For instance, health might be critiqued through the work of the famed sociologist Erving Goffman as a type of *stigmatizing rhetoric*, defined in moments of "mixed encounter" in which marks of difference based on size, color, or ability create groups of normals and, by exclusion, groups of others. From a Goffmanian perspective, affirmation of one's own health depends on the constant recognition, and indeed the creation, of the spoiled health of others.[7]

The work of the philosopher Ivan Illich similarly assists in critiquing health as a potentially *colonizing rhetoric*. Illich is arguably best known for his 1975 book *Medical Nemesis*, which argued that the medical establishment posed a "threat to health" through the production of clinical, social, and cultural "iatrogenesis."[8] In the 1980s, Illich expanded his critique to include the very definition of health itself. In a series of lectures titled "To Hell With Health," Illich bemoaned the negative effects of excessive preoccupation with health and the countless American industries that gained financially from promoting such preoccupation. "To hell with health," he is reported to have said. "It is the most cherished and destructive certitude of the modern world. It is a most destructive addiction." Illich did not mean that people need not seek relief from ailments and illnesses. Rather, he argued that American society promoted a definition of health based on an unattainable ideal, one that made no room for suffering, aging, dying, or other natural processes.[9]

So too, the scholarship of Talcott Parsons, Irving Zola, and a number of other medical sociologists casts health as a *normativizing rhetoric*. Zola, for instance, championed the phrase "temporarily abled bodies" as a way to challenge dominant notions of health, and critiqued the "socio-political consequences of medical influence" in determining matters of corporeality, ability, and, ultimately, normalcy.[10] And, of course, French sociologist Michel Foucault canonically promoted understanding health as a *discourse of power*, a discourse that is productive rather than repressive. From a Foucaultian perspective, American society's incessant talk about health produces and regulates itself and its subjects, while making it increasingly difficult to get outside of health. Such biopower subjugates utterances that we do not agree with and utterances that we do, both of which serve to remove us ever more from the possibility of real resistance.[11]

More recently, Adele Clarke, Peter Conrad, and a number of other academics and social critics demarcate health as a paradoxically *medicalizing rhetoric* that propagates various forms of medical profit or influence in an often inverse relation to human betterment. Early medicalization literature claimed that categories of health atherosclerotically narrowed when categories of disease expanded like an angioplastician's balloon. Clarke and colleagues track a more complex process of "biomedicalization" whereby biomedicine and technoscience conspire to define health as a moral obligation, a commodity, and a mark of status and self-worth. "In the biomedicalization era," they write, "the focus is no longer on illness, disability, and disease as matters of fate, but on health as a matter of ongoing moral self-transformation." Relatedly, public health scholar Deborah Lupton details ways in which public health policies "regulate" bodies by promoting definitions of health that represent "moral imperatives."[12]

Finally, growing numbers of practitioners from within medicine and public health, as well as members of patient activist groups, critique health as a problematically *consumerist rhetoric* that reflects social and economic norms under the guise of scientific information. In his erudite essay written in defense of smoking, musician and social activist Joe Jackson maligns anti-smoking "hysteria" through claims similar to ones that appear in this book. "We have become not only excessively reverent towards doctors and scientists, but increasingly willing to allow them to dictate our lifestyles and laws," Jackson writes. "Health is seen as an unqualified good. Who can be against 'health'?"[13] Meanwhile, physician H. Gilbert Welch argues that true health-care reform will only take place when America moves away from definitions of health that profit the "medical-industrial complex" of health professionals, pharmaceutical companies, biotechnology firms, manufacturers of diagnostic technologies, surgical centers, hospitals, and academic medical centers. "In the past, people sought health care because they were sick," Welch writes. "Now the medical-industrial complex seeks patients." In this system, "if health is the absence of abnormality, the only way to know you are healthy is to become a customer."[14]

Engagement with these and other critiques of health forces a set of questions central to the intentions of this book. Are present-day notions of health merely extensions of that-which-came-before, or are different forces at play in our current biopolitical age?[15] If the latter, then who are the new actors and agents? Who are the new victims and beneficiaries? Should the aim of critique be, as Illich once suggested, "liberation" from medical authority?[16] Or is medical authority even relevant in an era when pharmaceutical companies appeal directly to consumers, insurance companies set parameters of healthy living, and most people obtain medical information from infomercials, talk shows, package inserts, and the Internet?[17] What new selves and citizens are created by this health rhetoric, and what non-selves and non-citizens are constructed and then left out? Whose agendas are met by these new configurations, and whose are thwarted or replaced? Who are the new mortals, elitists, conservatives, liberals, structuralists, activists, and immigrants? And why?

This part, the theoretical part, comes relatively easily, and indeed any critique of health risks forming the very consensus that we are trying to work against. The much more difficult task is to ask what we should do about it. Where does a critique of health take us if we wish to be taken forward? What new possibilities and alliances arise? What new forms of activism or coalition can we create? What are our prospects for well-being? In short, what have we got if we ain't got health? Answering these "what to do" questions requires an emphasis on the concrete at the expense of the abstract, for if health is to be critiqued as too ideological a concept then surely we must hold resistance to this same standard. And address them we must, if we are not only to critique health, but to propose a viable set of alternatives.

What follows, then, is an attempt to distinguish a growing scholarly movement that regards health as a condition of ideology as well as longevity. Our analysis is in no way exhaustive, nor does it represent a uniform agenda of any sort. Rather, we highlight central lines of inquiry, debate, and even disagreement in an attempt to provoke further discussion. The authors represent opinion leaders from disciplines including medicine, law, bioethics, history, gender and LGBT studies, African American studies, disability studies, and literary studies, among others. Many of the chapters focus on constructions of health in the United States, although each author writes in awareness of the globalizing ways in which U.S. health is built on, and then often effaces, its connection to economies, clinical trials, lives, deaths, and side effects taking place beyond American shores. For the sake of overall coherence, each author has been asked to address the same question: *Why against health?*

The chapters appear in four thematic groupings, each of which addresses a specific avenue through which health is ideologically produced. Part I, "What Is Health, Anyway?" explores the basic problems involved in defining health. The section begins with a provocative challenge to modern-day notions of health by literary studies scholar Richard Klein. Taking his cue from Epicurean philosophers, Klein argues that present-day America is so strongly "in the clutches" of biomedical definitions of health that it loses sight of alternative approaches to well-being, namely those that emphasize the centrality of pleasure. Complicating Klein's celebration of indulgence, cultural theorist Lauren Berlant rejects seeing obesity as a disease of irresponsibility and focuses on two other factors: the exhausting effects of the laboring day and the mental health effects of eating to pause, to rest, and to suspend vigilance. Part I then concludes with medical anthropologist Vincanne Adams's critical analysis of the processes by which the notion of "health" in Global Health Sciences holds a tyrannical relationship to problems within the actual practices of global health.

Part II, "Seeing Health through Morality," considers the moral valences and assumptions embodied by particular constructions of health. Legal scholar Dorothy Roberts begins by unpacking the ways in which the rhetoric surrounding the production of pharmaceuticals designed to treat diseases in particular racial and ethnic groups stealthily supports a neoliberal shift of responsibility for public welfare from the state to the private realm of family and market. Communication studies scholar Kathleen LeBesco then presents a sharply contrasting view to Berlant's in Part I, arguing that the obesity epidemic is no epidemic at all, but rather an illustration of the "moral panic" surrounding a host of wider, cultural anxieties about identity, subjectivity, and rights. Finally, women's studies professor Joan Wolf explores medical and moral debates about whether breastfeeding is better than formula-feeding for babies. "I am not against health," Wolf writes, "but I am opposed to seemingly well-meaning advocates, including the government, presenting health as much simpler than it actually is."

Part III, "Making Health and Disease," anatomizes specific ways in which categories of health and illness are socially, historically, or politically produced. Chapters in this section particularly address how politics, corporate forces, special interests, and surprisingly shaky notions of consensus impact popular and medical definitions of mental health and its discontents. Bioethicist Carl Elliott critiques the shocking ways in which pharmaceutical company–driven marketing and propaganda campaigns shape psychiatric beliefs about disease. Literary scholar Christopher Lane then uses the strange, troubling history of passive-aggressive disorder to tell the story of how the number of official psychiatric diagnoses has "skyrocketed so dramatically that half the country is now said to suffer from at least one of them, and there's scarcely a quirk or trait left that couldn't be designated a new symptom." Cultural critic Lennard Davis tackles changing definitions of obsessive-compulsive disorder. Davis argues that psychiatry's exclusive focus on symptoms serves to flatten out understandings of mental distress. Anthropologist Joseph Masco concludes the section by shifting focus from clinical realms to political and historical ones. Masco adroitly shows how instant mass death, nuclear obliteration, and radiation-induced disease became normalized threats in the aftermath of the Second World War, producing new anxieties, new concepts of healthy life, and new relationships between citizens and the state.

Chapters in Part IV, "Pleasure and Pain after Health," actively refute or rearticulate basic formulations of health. Disability studies scholar Eunjung Kim's focus on individuals who understand their absence of sexual desire as an asexual identity or orientation, not as lack or dysfunction, leads to a broad discussion of the centrality of sexuality to Western notions of healthy bodies. Anthropologist S. Lochlann Jain then unpacks the paradoxes of cancer culture. Jain argues that marches for hope, research funding and direction, pharmaceutical interests, survivor rhetoric, and hospital advertisements overlap to form a broad hegemony that restricts the ways that cancer is talked about in the United States, while at the same time paradoxically constructing cancer as an individual problem, not a social or public one. Literature professor Tobin Siebers, also writing from the perspective of disability studies, then offers a political account of how pain triggers powerful emotions, opinions, and judgments. "I speak in the name of pain," Siebers explains, "to reveal that the fear of pain is one of the most pervasive and insidious justifications of disability oppression." Finally, legal theorist Anna Kirkland concludes *Against Health* by summarizing the book's main arguments and asking, "What next?"

Once again, this book's stand against health is not a stand against the authenticity of people's attempts to ward off suffering. We instead claim that individual strivings for health are, in some instances, rendered more difficult by the ways in which health is culturally configured and socially sustained. As we now turn to explore, health is a concept, a norm, and a set of bodily practices whose ideological work is often rendered invisible by the assumption that it is a monolithic, universal good. Sometimes, to be sure, this ideological function works for the betterment of many people by promoting herd immunity, longevity, happiness, or calm. Other times, ideology obfuscates the ways in which the good health of some persons depends on the ill health of others, or promotes purely political agendas under the guise of passion or concern. We hold that the conversations that doctors, patients, consumers, activists, pacifists, protesters, or policymakers have about health are enriched by recognizing that, when talking about health, they are not all talking about the same thing. And that articulating the disparate valences of "health" can lead to deeper, more productive, and indeed more healthy interactions about embodied expectations and intersubjective desires.

1. *Health*, April 2008; *Men's Health*, April 2008.

2. "Cialis (tadalafil): Official Site," Lilly USA, LLC, http://www.cialis.com/index. jsp, accessed 3/10/2008.

3. http://www.ezerex.com/?gclid=COi61uKA9JECFQLwPAodMic5wg, accessed 3/10/2008.

4. "Is This One of Yours?" Michigan Department of Community Health and the Michigan Association of Broadcasters, http://www.youtube.com/watch?v=mE-_zA-ZZIo; http://anti-smoking-ads.blogspot.com, accessed 3/10/2008.

5. Chad Terhune, "Lighten Up: Pepsi Sales Force Tries to Push 'Healthier' Snacks in Inner City," *Wall Street Journal*, October 5, 2006, A1.

6. We acknowledge, however, that more often the opposite association exists in capitalist societies. Wal-Mart Stores, Inc. grows more profitable by denying health care to its workers. And the stocks of tobacco corporations rise when the class action lawsuits of wronged individuals are thrown out of court, thereby allowing the production of more cigarettes. Inasmuch as Wal-Mart or tobacco shares rise in an inverse proportion to the health claims of workers or consumers, the health of economic bodies depends inversely on the health of individual ones.

7. Erving Goffman, *Stigma: Notes on the Management of Spoiled Identity* (Englewood Cliffs, NJ: Prentice Hall, 1963).

8. For Illich, Western medicine's conception of issues of healing, aging, and dying as medical illnesses effectively "medicalized" human life, rendering individuals and societies less able to deal with these "natural" processes. See his *Limits to Medicine: Medical Nemesis, the Expropriation of Health* (London: Marion Boyars, 1976). See also Renee C. Fox, "The Medicalization and Demedicalization of American Society," in *Doing Better and Feeling Worse: Health in the United States*, ed. John H. Knowles (New York: Norton, 1977); Peter Conrad, "The Discovery of Hyperkinesis: Notes on the Medicalization of Deviant Behavior," *Social Problems* 23, no. 1 (October 1975): 12–21; and Jonathan M. Metzl and Rebecca M. Herzig, "Medicalisation in the 21st Century: Introduction," *The Lancet* 369, no. 9562 (February 2007): 697–98.

9. See Lee Hoinacki and Carl Mitcham, eds., *The Challenges of Ivan Illich: A Collective Reflection* (Albany: State University of New York Press, 2002); see also "Ivan Illich at Penn State: Continuing the Conversation," Penn State University, http://www.pudel. uni-bremen.de/pdf/sym11_04_psu_en.pdf. Quotation from personal correspondence with Robert M. Duggan, February 28, 2007.

10. See Irving Zola, "In the Name of Health and Illness: On Some Socio-Political Consequences of Medical Influence," *Social Science and Medicine* 9, no. 2 (February 1975): 83–87. See also Irving Zola, "Bringing Our Bodies and Ourselves Back In: Reflections on a Past, Present, and Future 'Medical Sociology,'" *Journal of Health and Social Behavior* 32, no. 1 (March 1991): 1–16. We might also call on the work of the philosopher Louis Althusser to define health as an interpolating rhetoric that hails and defines patients and doctors both. This perspective helps deconstruct moments when, for instance, patients come to doctors' offices requesting advertised brand-name medications by name after having been hailed by drug advertisements. Such moments represent consumer empowerment, to be sure.

But the empowerment comes at the cost of entry into a symbolic order that precludes awareness of generics, herbal remedies, holistic medicines, and other alexiterics that are thereby metabolized as outside the economy of health.

11. See Michel Foucault, *The History of Sexuality* (New York: Pantheon, 1978).

12. Adele E. Clarke, Janet K. Shim, Laura Mamo, Jennifer Ruth Fosket, and Jennifer R. Fishman, "Biomedicalization: Technoscientific Transformations of Health, Illness, and U.S. Biomedicine," *American Sociological Review* 68, no. 2 (April 2003): 172. See also Peter Conrad, "Medicalization and Social Control," *Annual Review of Sociology* 18 (1992): 209–32; Deborah Lupton, *The Imperative of Health: Public Health and the Regulated Body* (New York: Sage, 1995).

13. Joe Jackson, "Smoke, Lies, and the Nanny State," http://www.joejackson.com/pdf/5smokingpdf_jj_smoke_lies.pdf, 3, accessed 9/7/2009.

14. H. Gilbert Welch, "To Overhaul the System, 'Health' Needs Redefining," *New York Times*, July 27, 2009, D5.

15. See, for example, John Dewey, *Theory of Valuation*, vol. 2, no. 4 of *International Encyclopedia of Unified Science*, ed. Otto Neurath (Chicago: University of Chicago Press, 1939), 1–67.

16. See Illich, *Limits*, 6–7.

17. See again Metzl and Herzig, "Medicalization," 697–98.

Part I

What Is Health, Anyway?

What Is Health and How Do You Get It?

RICHARD KLEIN

The title of this book, *Against Health*, arises out of the same counterintuitive impulse and obeys the same rhetorical strategy that led me to call two of my books *Cigarettes Are Sublime* and *Eat Fat*. I call that rhetorical strategy "contrarian hyperbole." When anything has been so debased or so glorified that its value is taken for granted, it becomes rhetorically necessary to exaggerate the value of its opposite in order for skepticism to be heard at all. With these books, I wanted to extol and celebrate the beauty of cigarettes and fat. This is not an easy task these days, when both substances have been vilified, burdened with intimations of disease and corruption. The truth, of course, is that they are not in themselves evil, but rather mixed blessings. Fat and cigarettes may be bad for your health, but they also dispense comfort, foster ease, and bestow beauty.

Similarly, the title of this book aims to contradict and contravene what is generally taken to be self-evident—to un-prize what is so highly prized these days in our public discourse and in our individual lives—the health to which we assign the highest value. Rarely do we even think of opposing health. To say we are "against health" is to utter a paradox, a sort of oxymoron in the Greek sense, from *oxus*, meaning "sharp," and *moros*, meaning "stupid." To be against health is to utter a sharp stupidity because, almost by definition, we cannot be against health. The very concept of health implies a positive value that one cannot but choose, as when Socrates argues that one can only choose the good. What is bad may be chosen only when it is a better evil, as in cutting off your arm to save your life.

Indeed, how can the value of health be demeaned when Aristotle makes it the entelechy, the very aim of all medicine? If to be against health is therefore stupid, or *moros*, it is also *oxus*, shrewd and terribly sharp. If we cannot logically be against it, we must be against certain uses of the word "health," or against the misuse of the concept itself. We can only be against "health" in scare quotes, "health" as it has been defined by a public discourse that reflects pharmaceutical, governmental, insurance, and media interests—not necessarily in that order.

In the United States, health has become a commodity and an industry. We spend vastly more than any other country on health care, and increasingly our health is our wealth. It is soon to replace manufacturing as the United States' principal economic engine. Nowhere in the world do people spend more resources to promote their health, and nowhere in the world are more people uninsured and thus without the means to pay for hospitalization. Forty-seven million people in the United States receive health care equivalent to that of third- and fourth-world societies.[1] In 2006, Americans spent about $35 billion on diets and diet services, in large part under the illusion that they were improving their health.[2] Yet we consistently fall beneath the United Kingdom, not to mention France, in every measure of public health. Some place American public health just above that of Slovenia.[3]

We may be nearing a point where the institutions of public health, the media, and commercial interests that surround it, and the ideological wisdom it dispenses, do more harm to the nation's health than good. The official version of health peddled by our current system is not only venal but potentially noxious. In some instances, public health has been transformed into a kind of iatric disease, a medically induced assault on the health of society. Our minders trumpet the obesity epidemic even as epidemiological evidence suggests that "yo-yo dieting" (repeatedly losing and regaining weight over a period of several years) actively damages the immune system.[4] At any given time, it is estimated that 50 percent of all women are on diets, and 95 percent of all diets fail. People obsessively diet in order to fight the obesity epidemic and constantly fail, as a result dying early from the repeated affronts to their metabolism induced by starving and binging. Indeed, the harmful effects of weight cycling may be equal to the risk of simply remaining obese, which also doubles the chance of early death.[5] It appears that the epidemic of dieting may actually be worse for our health than the obesity epidemic. In fact, fewer than 26,000 people a year die of being overweight, down from 400,000, according to the latest information.[6] The more we diet, the fatter we seem to become. In the spirit of this volume, I don't think we should necessarily conclude that dieting is riskier than obesity. But the mere possibility calls us to be suspicious of the claim we have been persuaded to believe, namely that obesity is riskier than obsessive dieting or diet drugs.

To be against health, therefore, is to be critical of the myths and lies concerning our health that are circulated by the media and paid for by large industries. It is to demystify their hidden moralizing and their political agenda, exposing what we might properly call the current ideology of health. Such a move or movement requires submitting particular epidemiological claims to skeptical critique, denouncing the misuses of that science and its extension into social policy where its conclusions are highly subject to doubt or refutation.[7] It also means expanding the idea of iatric disease to include the moral and physical harm that is done to the public by particular nostrums of public health, particularly those that impose constraints and privations "for your own good," as the saying goes.[8] My concern is with the particular ways in which public health is used for moral edification and as an instrument of social control with political implications for individual freedom.

In 1993, I wrote:

> The passionate excess of zeal with which cigarettes are everywhere stig-
> matized may signal that some more pervasive, subterranean, and danger-
> ous passions are loose that directly threaten our freedom. The freedom to
> smoke ought to be understood as a significant token of the class of free-
> doms, and when it is threatened one should look instantly for what other
> controls are being tightened, for what other checks on freedom are being
> administered.[9]

In retrospect, my claim seems prophetic of the increasing tendency of government to regulate our pleasure, our food, and our private behavior, even as its power grows more intrusive and more repressive of our civil liberties and our public habits. The dictation of personal health and hygiene by the state is a common feature of theocracies and totalitarian states. Hitler banned smoking out of concerns for public health and personal purity. In the name of health, political and sectarian repression is often at work.

The deconstruction of health seeks to pursue evidence that what is systematically tabooed and banned in both formal and informal wars against drugs and disease are substances and conditions that have distinct characteristics, different personalities, so to speak, with diverse roles in social history. Many such substances have social and medical benefits that are ignored or minimized.[10]

As I see it, *Against Health* proclaims a critical task, a great deconstructive act of mining and displacing the presumably solid foundations of the social institution of Health in order to question its most basic assumptions. But, like every proper deconstruction, being against health implies the further necessity of putting forth an alternative idea of health, a term that we can no longer use, but one that we can hardly do without.

I hold that we are so strongly in the clutches of Health with a capital "H" that we lose sight of definitions and concepts other than those widely advertised and promoted. In what follows, I attempt to think outside of Health by proposing an alternative approach to well-being. My conceptualization takes its cue from a long line of Epicurean philosophers, beginning with the fourth-century b.c. philosopher who founded his "Garden" in Athens, close by the Platonic Academy. The Garden of Epicurus has inspired many adherents to its teachings, including the poet Horace in Roman times and later Pierre Gassendi, François Bernier, Charles de Saint-Évremond, Ninon de l'Enclos, Denis Diderot, Jeremy Bentham, and Friedrich Nietzsche. Thomas Jefferson referred to himself as an Epicurean.

Let me give you a quick example of an alternative idea of health. You may not have heard of Ninon de l'Enclos. One of the greatest courtesans in the court of Louis XIII, she slept with royals and the most desirable men in the realm, conducted the most brilliant salon, and wrote the wittiest philosophical letters to ever speak about the nature of love. She was a great reader of Epicurus and his disciple Montaigne. In the eighth of her *Letters to the Marquis de Sévigné*, "The necessity for love and its primitive cause," de l'Enclos writes:

> What would vigorous youth be without love? A long illness—it would not be existence; it would be vegetating. Love is to our hearts what winds are to the sea. They grow into tempests, true; they are sometimes even the cause of shipwrecks. But the winds render the sea navigable, their constant agitation of its surface is the cause of its preservation, and if they are often dangerous, it is for the pilot to know how to navigate in safety.

According to de l'Enclos, if a life in the best of vigorous health is without love, it is no life at all, only a long illness. Even health is illness without love; conversely, there is no illness that love cannot cure or make tolerable. At the same time, love is trouble. Like wind, it troubles the surface of the sea, but it also makes navigation possible. The agitation of love preserves the self, keeps it healthy even when—especially when—it is sick. The risk of love, which so often ends in shipwreck, is what keeps a person healthy.

But there are other classic paths to health. Socrates believed in dancing every morning. We could do more for public health if the government spent a fraction of what it spends curbing smoking on promoting dancing. An Epicurean approach asks not what temptations need to be avoided in the name of health. Instead it asks, "What is health, and how do you get it?" An Epicurean perspective is first critical, initiating the critique of health by asking what it is good for. But it does not shrink from the next question: "What view of health are we for?" Is there an alternative to public policy that promotes Health?

Imagine another world in which public policy declared that pleasure is the principal means to health. The very idea of pleasure, if one can speak of it in the singular and not the plural (is there something all pleasures have in common?), comprises the most diverse and even contradictory notions. Of these, the most clearly contradictory is the paradox of what Burke or Kant or Freud call "negative pleasure," which is understood to underlie forms of masochism and the experience of the sublime. In Kant's *Critique of Judgment*, the sublime always entails a negative moment of shock or fearful awe as one component of its greater good feeling, its aesthetic pleasure. Leaving aside these antinomies, can we agree to call pleasure both the slow, economic accumulation of delicious tension and its abrupt and self-vacating explosion of release?[11] This is the distinction the French make between *plaisir* and *jouissance*, between two different types of pleasure. But let us for the moment overlook these distinctions that will eventually need to be preserved and analyzed.

The promotion of Epicurean pleasures seeks to emulate Bartolomeo Platina, the great fifteenth-century scholar, papal librarian, and Epicurean who wrote *De honesta voluptate et valetudine* (On Honest Pleasure and Good Health) while imprisoned in the castle San Angelo in Rome where a vengeful Pope Paul II had thrown him. He starts from the classical Epicurean premise that pleasure is not only a positive value but the highest value and that health is its necessary supplement. A person cannot be sick, and still feel good. She cannot be depressed, or physically debauched from alcohol and drugs, say, and still have pleasurable feelings. Following Platina and his master Epicurus, however, the corollary is also true. Not only is health the *sine qua non* of pleasure (that without which there is none), but pleasure improves your health. Put another way, if you inhibit the body's pleasure, you provoke disease.

Over the gates to his Garden (it was not a school), Epicurus inscribed the hedonist creed: "Stranger, here you will do well to tarry; here our highest good is pleasure." With an eye to what was fitting and measured and moderate, Epicurus indulged his senses. After all, he believed that excessive pleasure, like stoic privation, ruins one's health and weakens the will. Thomas Jefferson, himself a hedonist, agreed. In 1819, he wrote to William Short, saying that "the doctrine of Epicurus . . . is the most rational system remaining of the philosophy of the ancients, as frugal of vicious indulgence and fruitful of virtue as the hyperbolical extravagances of his rival sects."[12]

Recently, it has become un-American to be Epicurean, to consider pleasure, even moderately indulged, to be the highest good. An old strain of

American Puritanism to which Jefferson was immune, if not allergic, has become the new morality. Dressing itself up in the language of public health, this new morality views the least indulgence in adult pleasure as the sign of a nascent habit on the way to becoming a dangerous compulsion. In a sense, of course, that is precisely what distinguishes adult pleasures from childish ones: adult pleasures can quickly become habitual. But without risk, there is no adult pleasure, and risk is what keeps us alive, not just living on. Perhaps that is why every single person I know has been addicted—habituated to something—at some time in life and has had a problem dealing with it. It is an all but inevitable consequence of the pleasures we seek, particularly in America, where we are publicly spurred on to consume by advertisements and stresses that excite desire. It is not all bad. Nietzsche says that nothing in life is better than our habits, as long as they don't perdure. "I love brief habits," he writes, "and consider them an inestimable means for getting to know many things and states, down to the bottom of their sweetness and bitternesses."[13]

Each of us would like to know how to draw the fine line between the moderation Epicurus practiced and the intemperance he deplored. In *On Honest Pleasure and Good Health*, Platina writes, "Not all foods suit all people. . . . To my mind, no one eats what fills him with distaste, or harms, or pains, or kills." Platina is referring specifically to eating, but his suggestion can be taken more generally: we each consume what our body or spirit craves. You may only require one drink a day to ease your arteries, whereas I may need two or three. But when I start to need three or four a day, I'm probably getting into trouble. And if it isn't martinis at lunch that get me in trouble, it could be the cigarettes I sneak in the garage, or the poker game I lose twice a week, or the attractive babysitter, or the alluring congressional page. (What makes babysitters so irresistibly attractive, I have often thought, is their being simultaneously nubile children and caring mothers; the same may be true of congressional pages.) It belongs to the very nature of adult pleasure that it has the potential for getting out of hand. If it did not entail the risk of being immoderate, the pleasure it procures would lose its intensity.

For many people, a life without the oil of drink becomes too much to bear. A little wine eases the vague and subcutaneous unease that stress puts on our muscles; a martini induces a moment of forgetfulness when the anxieties and fears of the day recede. In pursuit of happiness, Americans are insistently encouraged to consume vast quantities of anti-anxiety drugs and antidepressants, but booze is never publicly celebrated.

Take, for example, a recent report issued by the National Center on Addiction and Substance Abuse (CASA) at Columbia University that describes alcohol as "a premier drug of abuse in America."[14] Stigmatizing alcohol as a drug is like calling the perfume Chanel No. 5 a chemical. (It too can be addictive.) Nowhere in the report do its authors reflect on the charms and benefits of alcohol, on the sociability it has promoted from the dawn of time, on the pleasure and consolation it has infused into the lives of billions over the course of human history. Nowhere do the authors consider the possibility that alcohol may be necessary for the very existence of human civilization, since, as far as we know, the consumption of fermented beverages coincides with its origins. Without alcohol's sweet poison, there may not have been any civilization at all, and without civilization, as Woody Allen once noted, we would never have had the Ice Capades.

Even when epidemiology is not manipulated to serve special interests, it tells the truth of an aggregate. By definition, epidemiology says nothing about a particular person's mortal destiny or the health that accompanies it. An Epicurean view of health focuses not on what makes us identical to the scientists' cohort, but what makes each of us irreducible singularities. Each one of us is a throw of the genetic and historical dice, born into this world with peculiar strengths and weaknesses, and with the singular obligation to take responsibility for our individual health. In short, health for the Epicurean is more a matter of art than of science, more an aesthetic than a biological question. Each of us has to find his or her own road to health. This takes cunning and, these days, some scientific curiosity. For an Epicurean, the first curiosity is about our body—how it works, how it responds to pleasure and pain.

In *The Physiology of Taste*, the nineteenth-century Epicurean Jean Anthelme Brillat-Savarin wrote: "When we eat, we receive a certain indefinable and peculiar impression of happiness originating in instinctive consciousness. When we eat, too, we repair our losses and prolong our lives."[15] Pleasure may thus be a form of intelligence, an intuitive science as well as an art. Some nations have more of this intelligence than others. As M.F.K. Fisher writes in *The Art of Eating*, "France eats more consciously, more intelligently than any other nation."[16] There are serious scientists who believe in the French paradox, that the gourmand's steady diet of foie gras and good red wine protects him from risk of heart disease. Michel Montignac, the French Dr. Atkins, believes in the healthful, slimming virtues of protein and fat but also recommends the purifying and invigorating powers of good French wine—advice the French hardly need, having heartily drunk their wine since Rabelais.[17]

Whenever anyone asked Julia Child to name her guilty pleasures, she responded, "I don't have any guilt." Epicureanism not only absolves us of guilt, it says that our guilty pleasures might actually be keeping us healthy—

mentally, physically, or both. Like Proust, the doctor's son, we might even consider it perversely healthy to sacrifice our health in order to write the greatest novel of the century. Julia Child was vigorous into her nineties not despite slathering chickens with butter, but because of it. Only you can judge, however, what your body needs and what gives you pleasure. It may be vital to know that cigarettes are bad for your health, but you might at the same time feel, like Sartre, that "Life without cigarettes is worthless."

In America, we have become strangely divorced from our bodies, counting calories on every product in the supermarket, watching blood pressure, measuring cholesterol, and sacrificing pleasure for prurience. These days, we do not eat for pleasure, but to lower our numbers. Yet we are one of the fattest nations in the world and growing every day more obese. But what do we stand to lose if we lose the enjoyment and pleasure that we derive from good eating and drinking? We may stand to lose everything. The epidemiologist cannot tell us what the Epicurean wants to know: What should I choose to love without guilt? What is good for me? What keeps me happy? What, in the best sense, keeps me healthy?

The New Epicureanism

In certain European philosophical circles, there has been a recent spike of interest in Epicurus, and not only among Marxists. (Marx wrote his doctoral thesis on Epicurus.) Like every Greek, Epicurus was obliged to believe in the pantheon of Greek gods who lived on Mount Olympus; but he did so without having to suppose that these gods were even remotely interested in human affairs. As a result, Epicurus needed to find principles for living that were based not on theological, but on materialist (or, we might say, scientific) conceptions of the world—those which explained all nature, including mind and spirit, with reference not to the supernatural, but to harmonies and atomic processes. Marx studied Epicurus because the Greek philosopher was the great ancient popularizer of the earlier materialist philosophers Lucippus and Democritus, who, in the fourth and fifth centuries b.c., were the first to propound an atomistic doctrine. Epicurus in turn directly influenced the Roman Lucretius, whose *De rerum natura* became the authority for Renaissance materialism and the basis of the whole philosophical tradition that runs from Bacon to Locke to Hume and Hobbes and all the way to Feuerbach, who thought that "you are what you eat."

Neo-Epicureans argue that the entire philosophical tradition since Plato— perhaps philosophy itself—has always rejected materialism and has forever been in love with idealism. Even the so-called materialist philosophies exhibit forms of Platonic idealism; this idealism may be turned on its head, as it were, but its articulations are still in place. The new, radical Epicureanism, on the other hand, is non-philosophical. It is a new way of articulating the relation between theory and practice; it is a praxis of thinking about pleasure and its value, in and of itself, as well as from the standpoint of health. Like Nietzsche, the Epicurean does not aspire to negate philosophy for that would only be another way of affirming it. Philosophy is nothing but the history of its successive negations. Rather, Epicurus teaches us how to look away from the tradition. "Looking up and away shall be my only negation," Nietzsche asserts in *The Gay Science*.[18] Like Nietzsche, neo-Epicureans start their thinking not with ideas but with what Epicurus insists is the origin of thought, the body.

Broadly put, neo-Epicureans suppose not only that you are what you eat, but that you think what you eat. Take German idealism, says Nietzsche. It has the leaden consistency and gaseous redolence of a diet thick with potatoes. Italian thought, one might add, is marked by the slippery texture and doughy blandness of pasta. Jewish metaphysics has the astringency and smoky intensity of briny pickles and cured fish. The indistinctness of Buddhist thought resembles white rice. Neo-Epicureans aim to discover not just a philosophy of being, but a hygiene for living, not a universal system, but a way of thinking about good health in terms of the peculiar proclivities of the individual body.

In the historical debate between mind and matter, mind won and silenced the voice of the body; it interpreted the body in terms of mind and considered it a mute machine that only reason could discover. It is time to recover that corporeal voice, to recast the Epicurean thinking that puts pleasure in the place of thought, that imagines bodily pleasure to be a kind of thinking. Good health will then be understood as a consequence of good pleasure, and adult pleasure will be prized, not tabooed, moderated not censored, indulged not feared.

NOTES

1. Tony Pugh, "Number of Americans without Health Insurance Hits New High," *McClatchey*, August 28, 2007, http://www.mcclatchydc.com/homepage/story/19319.html.

2. Melissa McNamara, "Diet Industry Is Big Business: Americans Spend Billions on Weight-Loss Products Not Regulated by the Government," *CBS Evening News*, December 1, 2006, http://www.cbsnews.com/stories/2006/12/01/eveningnews/main2222867.shtml.http://www.cbsnews.com/sections/eveningnews/eyeontech/main501464.shtml.

3. World Health Organization, "World Health Organization Assesses the World's Health Systems," June 21, 2000, http://www.who.int/whr/2000/media_centre/press_release/en/index.html.

4. John O'Neil, "VITAL SIGNS: BEHAVIOR; The Dangers of Yo-Yo Dieting," *New York Times*, June 8, 2004, http://www.nytimes.com/2004/06/08/health/vital-signs-behavior-the-dangers-of-yo-yo-dieting.html?sec=health.

5. "Maintaining Weight Lost," The Yale Medical Group, October 2005. See also P. Ernsberger and R. J. Koletsky, "Weight Cycling," *JAMA: Journal of the American Medical Association* 273, no. 13 (1995): 998–99.

6. Katherine M. Flegal, Barry I. Graubard, David F. Williamson, and Mitchell H. Gail, "Excess Deaths Associated with Underweight, Overweight, and Obesity," *JAMA: Journal of the American Medical Association* 293, no. 15 (2005): 1861–67. See also Gina Kolata, "Data on Deaths from Obesity Is Inflated, U.S. Agency Says," *New York Times*, October 5, 2007, http://www.nytimes.com/2004/11/24/health/24obese.html. See also "Genes Take Charge, and Diets Fall by the Wayside," *New York Times*, May 8, 2007, http://www.nytimes.com/2007/05/08/health/08fat.html.

7. Cf. Michael Ward and Jan Wright, *The Obesity Epidemic* (New York: Routledge, 2005), 11. Cf. also Gina Kolata, *Rethinking Thin: The New Science of Weight Loss—and the Myths and Realities of Dieting* (New York: Farrar, Straus and Giroux 2007).

8. Jacob Sullum, *For Your Own Good* (New York: Free Press, 1998).

9. Richard Klein, *Cigarettes Are Sublime* (Durham: Duke University Press, 1993), 15.

10. I like to keep track of all the positive medical virtues that researchers are forever finding in substances and conditions that are officially reviled or demeaned. This list does not even mention all the positive advantages one derives of a different sort. Moderate drinking seems to be good for the heart and circulatory system, and it probably protects against type 2 diabetes and gallstones. More than 100 prospective studies show an inverse association between moderate drinking and risk of heart attack, ischemic (clot-caused) stroke, peripheral vascular disease, sudden cardiac death, and death from all cardiovascular causes. (See Harvard School of Public Health, "Alcohol: Balancing Risks and Benefits," http://www.hsph.harvard.edu/nutritionsource/what-should-you-eat/alcohol-full-story/index.html.)

Results of studies at Palermo suggest an inverse association between smoking cigarettes, coffee drinking, and alcohol consumption and the incidence of Parkinson's disease. In addition, the more coffee you drink, the more it protects the liver from the effects of alcohol. (See E. K. Tan, C. Tan, S. M. Fook-Chong, S. Y. Lum et al., "Dose-dependent Protective Effect of Coffee, Tea, and Smoking in Parkinson's Disease: A Study in Ethnic Chinese," *Journal of Neurological Science* 216, no. 1 (December 15, 2003): 163–67.)

Coffee, if you were not aware, is the new panacea. Scientists in Lisbon report that caffeine intake was associated with a significantly lower risk of Alzheimer's disease, independently of other potentially confounding variables. Studies in Berlin suggest that the use of non-steroidal anti-inflammatory drugs (like ibuprofen), wine, and coffee consumption, and regular physical activity may delay the onset of Alzheimer's disease or reduce its rate of progression. Researchers in Sweden assert that the findings of a recent study support the hypothesis that coffee consumption protects against diabetes in women. Who needs health insurance when we have Starbucks on every corner? (See also "Cup of Coffee a Day

Could Help Protect Against Alzheimer's Disease, Study Suggests," *Science Daily*, April 3, 2008, http://www.sciencedaily.com/releases/2008/04/080402194407.htm.)
These facts remind me of the moment in Woody Allen's film *Sleeper* when, after a long hibernation, Miles Monroe wakes up in the year 2500 and doctors rush to give him coffee, cigarettes, and chocolate. As we learned from Debra Waterhouse's book *Why Women Need Chocolate* (Darby, PA: Diane Publishing, 1993), for reasons that are hormonal, metabolic, and moral, all women need the equivalent of a Hershey's kiss every day at four o'clock. My wife needs a Klein kiss at least once a day.

11. Sigmund Freud, *The Standard Edition of the Complete Psychological Works of Sigmund Freud*, 24 vols., trans. James Strachey, Anna Freud, Alix Strachey, and Alan Tyson (London: Hogarth Press and the Institute of Psycho-Analysis, 1953–74), 18: 9.

12. Thomas Jefferson, "Letter to William Short," Epicurous.info, http://www.epicurus.info/etexts/Jefferson.html.

13. Friedrich Nietzsche, *The Gay Science* (New York: Vintage Press, 1974) 295.

14. *JAMA*, February 2, 2004, p. 18.

15. Jean Anthelme Brillat-Savarin, *M.F.K. Fisher's Translation of the Physiology of Taste: or, Meditations on Transcendental Gastronomy* (*New York*: Harcourt Brace Jovanovich, 1978), 46.

16. M.F.K. Fisher and Joan Reardon, *The Art of Eating* (Hoboken, NJ: Wiley, 2004), 15.

17. Michel Montignac, *Eat Yourself Thin* (Paris: Montignac Publishing, 2004).

18. Nietzsche, *The Gay Science*, 36.

Risky Bigness

On Obesity, Eating, and
the Ambiguity of "Health"

LAUREN BERLANT

I'm not against health at all, not even a little. But in a time of massive obesity *and* starvation, food plenty *and* food shortage, health isn't what it used to be. This chapter is about the obesity epidemic, and the relation of risky bigness to what it *feels like* to eat. My claim is that physical health and mental health are duking it out these days and, as a parent says to warring siblings, *somebody's going to get hurt*. Somebody's already hurt, actually. The obesity epidemic is widely understood to threaten not just all consumers of Western junk food, but particularly the poor and, in the United States at least, the non-white. This is not only a problem for individuals but a symptom of something askew for entire populations.

What follows is a different kind of explanation for the epidemic of overfeeding that has engendered "obesity" as a word we hear every day. It will not demonize bad habits or individual failures of will, nor cast a conspiratorial gaze at some "obesity industrial complex" for duping people into eating bad, bad foods. It will not argue that people need more "education." It will also not make a "pro-fat acceptance" argument, although I am entirely on the side of eliminating bodily stigma.

To many these days, the obese body serves as a billboard advert for impending sickness and death. But this chapter considers obesity as an effect of people's *attachment to life*. Instead of seeing obesity as a disease of the will or as simple irresponsibility, it looks at how exhaustion shapes the reproduction of life at home and at work. This massive and spreading fatigue has changed fundamentally our relation to eating, which is a different topic than our relation to food. I argue that eating provides a kind of rest for the exhausted self, an interruption of being good, conscious, and intentional that feels like a relief. This rejuvenating function has almost nothing to do with the relative goodness or badness of what one eats, or how. We are now caught in a competition between kinds of health. How can that be?

The contemporary human is fatigued in the literal sense but also a metaphorical one, as in what metal "feels" when it no longer can bear the stress placed on it. I will suggest that eating is like the "self-medicating" practices of drinking, sex, television, sports fandom, video games, and drugs, but not because they're addictive. (This varies, after all.) My claim is that these kinds of activities provide opportunities to become absorbed in the present, opportunities that suffuse people with the pleasure of engaged appetites and enable people to *feel* more resilient in the everyday. This sense of resilience is different from actual resilience: bodies wear out from the pleasures that help them live on. But the growth of the appetite industries in a world where there is less time to enjoy them says something of the desperate need for relief provided by the pleasures that make it possible to get up tomorrow and do it all over again. We will learn nothing about how to cure self-induced ill health from appetitive excess if we don't understand its mental health function. Sure, addictive behavior is associated with depression: but it also discharges stress. Legislating more consciousness won't fix it. Shaming patients won't fix it: they've already learned to dread "health" as a pleasure buzzkill. Knowledge is not really power where the appetites are concerned.

So, I am claiming that this is a better way to think about the rising tide of unhealthy fatness in the United States and Europe. People are tired from work, tired from being good, tired from being overwhelmed by the demands of production and the reproduction of life. Eating can perform a kind of irresponsibility that's mostly not exuberant (although sometimes "being bad" is a form of minor triumph) but folds a vitalizing pleasure into the spaces of ordinary living. Obesity is an effect of the intensity with which so many people need more and more mental health vacations from their exhaustion. I will close by claiming that any policy advancing more consciousness and intention where eating and the appetites are concerned neglects the place of the rejuvenating pleasures in the maintenance of everyday life. Mental health vacations are beating out the physical virtues, and if this is not an unmixed good, it might be a necessity.

Thus, if the obesity epidemic is a symptom of something, it is not just one motivating thing. What is a symptom? A symptom is a fiction the body develops to tell you that a process that you *can't see* is awry. Obesity and eating in everyday life are not just symptoms of something off in individuals. They also point to social problems in maintaining equilibrium and optimism in everyday life. This has something to do with work and leisure and how hard it is to generate an enduring sense of well-being. This is why the pleasure people take in "letting themselves go" might be a pleasure that's both for *and* against health.

My thought about this began with a beautiful idea of the geographer David Harvey. Harvey writes fabulously polemical books about how globalization affects people's visceral lives. In *Spaces of Hope*, Harvey writes that under capitalism sickness is defined as the inability to work.[1] When I first read that thought, I could not breathe in the face of its profound truth. Then I thought about Sudafed commercials. Sudafed is a drug that suppresses headcold symptoms that cause difficulties in breathing. The commercials for it are never about *curing* ill health, though: they're about managing symptoms so that cold sufferers can go to work while ill, while infectious and infected. The drug is not about getting better, moving toward health, but about treading water, maintaining income and momentum. It is about sacrificing one domain of well-being for health in a few others, namely the economic and emotional. Likewise, many arguments for exercise and healthy eating do not focus on cultivating better health: they're about having more energy to be more productive.

Harvey was sharing an open secret about contemporary life: it's overwhelming. Not only must we work to live, but we must do whatever we need to do, including stay sick, in order to work. Harvey's is not the whole story of capitalism's effect on health in the "developed world," but let's stay awhile with this part of it. He points out that Marx predicted today's labor-related erosion of our bodily fortitude. Consider the physical and mental tasks any worker faces to become used to the demands of technology and routine. Everyone has to produce energy and develop skills for physical, mental, and emotional labor, skills that have to appear to be part of the body's hardwiring. All of these domains of competence demand energy from workers, wherever they are in the hierarchy of class privilege. Think of any worker's accommodations to the rhythms of acceptable hunger and timed breaks within confining work environments that are often both under- and overwhelming. Think of the energy it takes to manage the sociality of lunch and rest along with giving the body what it needs. Think about the ways energy drinks, sugar, and caffeine fuel the process of simply getting by. Think about the imperative to focus amidst distraction, and the imperative to stay in a decent mood. Working the workday requires fatigue management and mood management, efficiency, and affective labor at work and later at home. The project of being reliable to the economic system that ostensibly supports you (while you're supporting it) therefore choreographs not only your skills but your physical, cognitive, and emotional energy. Not only that, it shapes how you *imagine* the everyday life of competence, satisfaction, and happiness. The conditions of the reproduction of life shape fantasy itself: one's optimism for living, one's pragmatism about what it takes, and what it would mean not to be sapped by all that. I'm not saying that we are *determined* by the scene of labor, or only miserable in it—not at all—but rather that our bodily lives are shaped pretty significantly by its demands.

Political theorists often phrase this kind of discussion about how citizens experience time, embodiment, consciousness, intention, and action in terms of the concept of *sovereignty*. The sovereign man is not, in theory, a dependent one: he thinks, intends, acts, and has effects. He has a will that shapes life and death, and he uses it; not only that, but he feels it. To have sovereignty is to *feel* sovereign. One's power is identical to one's sense of power. The individual is like a nation, in control over the conditions of life. In fact, democratic nations are supposed to protect the sovereignty of citizens over their everyday lives. One kind of sovereignty secures another. This fantasy of sovereignty produces paranoia as its security force: it posits any potential loss of control as a threat from something *outside*. What's outside threatens to diminish one's sovereignty over one's own personal and political life: as though one had sovereignty over one's own life.

When I call sovereignty a fantasy, I don't mean to demean fantasy. But we were never sovereign. Governors are acting sovereign when they save someone from being put to death. The police are sovereign by proxy when they decide whether or not to arrest you. You may feel sovereign when you make decisions, like obeying a stop sign or protesting, but by then the sense of sovereignty has become something else, a measure of compliance. In short, usually one's sense of autonomy in sovereignty is limited at best, and often points to an unclear situation. We remember the acts we did that we identify with as sovereign acts, producing effects we like, and we forget almost everything else; we also, at the same time, seek to limit our sovereignty by seeking out collaborative relations with all sorts of people, institutions, and governments. We accommodate strangers, intimates, and colleagues, and we expect (if things are just) to be accommodated. We want to accommodate except when we don't; we want to feel free *from* except when we want to feel free *for* and free *with*. Sometimes we like having no control and being unconscious. Usually, we throw ourselves into things without thinking much, and then we want that to work out well.

Thus, the idea that we should be organizing the world around increasing sovereignty in order to diminish irrationality and reduce vulnerability means that we are being governed by a fantasy that denies other things about how we live. We know that relations of dependency and care are not just concessions but emotional necessities. We know that reciprocity matters in financial and emotional economies, that the concept of trust is both affective and economic. We know that modes of kinship that derive from relations of care are not just normative obligations but foundations for whatever good life we imagine. We know that we act habitually and impulsively all the time, and that life would be unimaginable if we were actually forced to decide consciously at every minute, if we were hypervigilant about matters of life and death like movie monsters waiting to be crossed. This is why I think that, when it comes to appetitive disorders, the discourse of responsibility and consciousness fights against the contradictions and vagaries of how humans must actually operate. This doesn't mean that we're doomed to chaos all the time, either. But we must begin thinking about how to survive and thrive not by imagining people in the tableau of their greatest self-conscious control but by seeing the patterns of activity that at once advance and contradict survival in light of the pressures of contemporary everyday life. Then we need to rethink everyday life.

All of this juggling of actual social involvement and phantasmatic sovereignty takes place in the context of everyday lives that are maximally stressed out. This is to say that the work of getting through the day exhausts our *practical sovereignty*. We are compelled to act responsibly. That is what it means to be competent, an adult. The obesity epidemic, part of the expansion of the physical unhealth we see everywhere, is a symptom of our struggle to survive the day, the week, the month, and the life, an *as-if sovereignty* that depletes resources of compliance from us that we barely have. The stress we experience in environments that are already absorbing the best part of our energy and creativity is so enormous that we are forced to ask whether we can even *imagine* this world as a world organized for health. If not, perhaps it is our fantasy of the good life that needs reparative attention personally, mass culturally, and politically.

The evidence is stark that this symptom of stressed-out bodies and lives pervades the entire world economy. The obesity or "globesity" phenomenon is sweeping the United States as well as the whole Westernizing world.[2] In the contemporary U.S. context, it is motivated not so much by doctors but by insurance companies, health departments, and corporate public relations offices. If this chapter were a living organism, its footnotes would expand daily from a diet of crisis-and-response headlines in mainstream and professional papers, journals, newspapers, and magazines. The first time I presented this chapter as a talk, the morning headlines heralded a crisis for Kraft Foods, whose profit was depressed by a fall in the rate of increase in Oreo sales and only partially stemmed by real gains in the equally unhealthy breakfast (pseudo)health bar market; the next time I presented this chapter, they broadcast news of a hastily written "cheeseburger bill," introduced in the Congress to protect companies from litigation stemming from charges that corporate food produced obesity-inducing addiction (this bill was passed as the "Personal Responsibility in Food Consumption Act of 2005");[3] the third time I presented this chapter, I was greeted by an AOL headline, "Would You Like a Serving of Obesity with That?" which talked about a voluntary trend toward putting nutrition labels on the menus of franchise restaurants; and on the morning of a recent revision, an article appeared in the *New York Times* stating that the French fry is now the most frequently and voluminously eaten vegetable by all children in the United States over fifteen months old, an article soon succeeded by a controversial claim that childhood consumption of French fries leads to increased incidence of adult breast cancer.[4]

In short, one thing that the obesity epidemic is, is a media effect. Some people even talk about it cynically as an orchestrated incitement to sell drugs, services, and newspapers, and to justify new governmental and medical oversight on the populations whose appetites are out of control (a conventional view of the masses, subalterns, the sexual, and so on).[5] Cynicism makes some sense: we learned most recently from AIDS, after all, that the epidemic concept is not a neutral description, but always a contribution to ongoing mechanisms of social distinction. Who's degenerate, who's competent, and who's out of and in control? Is being seriously overweight a personality flaw or a disease? Is adding stress to the healthcare system from the stress of everyday life the same as incompetence in social membership, citizenship, or personhood itself? How we answer these questions shapes the imaginable and pragmatic logics of "cure."

So, how best to characterize this object, our scene, our case? We know that "the obesity epidemic" unduly burdens the working classes of the contemporary United States, the United Kingdom and, increasingly, all countries in which there is heavy participation in the global processed-food regime. Scientific and journalistic studies recite the phrases in scandalized disbelief: "The number of extremely obese American adults—those who are at least 100 pounds overweight" or with a Body Mass Index of 50 "has quadrupled since the 1980s" and . . . works out to 1 in every 50 adults."[6] Likewise, the slightly less obese percentages (BMI of 40 or over) grew to 1 in 40, and the percentage of ordinary overweight grew to 1 in 5. The problem requires no rhetorical hyperbole to match its actual scale. For the first time in the history of the world there are as many overfed as underfed people, and for the first time in the history of the world the overfed are no longer the wealthiest compared to the poor and starving.[7] All Americans, the absolutely and relatively well off as well as the poor, are getting fatter. But it is specifically the bodies of U.S. working-class and subproletarian populations that weaken most intensively from the pressure of obesity on their organs and skeletons. Meanwhile, U.S. and corporate food policy continues to emaciate drastically the land and the bodies of our food producers to the south, in Mexico and South America, as well as those in Africa and rural China.[8]

This inversion is more than an irony or a paradox: mass emaciation and obesity are mirror symptoms of the malnourishment of the poor throughout the contemporary world. But how does the recognition of the contours of a case organize our imagination in responding to it? We understand the need to get food to the underfed poor, and quickly, for that is what they would do if they had the means of production in their hands. As for the overfed, owning the means of production might well produce more overfeeding, more exercise of agency toward death and unhealth, and certainly not against power. Unless one wants to see being overweight as a protest against "elite" notions of health and wealth, there is nothing promising, heroic, or critical about this development.[9]

Long-term problems of embodiment within capitalism, in the zoning of the everyday and the work of getting through it, are less successfully addressed in the typical temporalities of crisis. How else, then, to understand the intersection of the long history of poor people's shorter lives and the particular conditions of contemporary speed-up—people working harder and longer just to keep afloat? What does it mean for thinking about the ethics of longevity when we consider the consequences of work and sickness in an unequal health system, when, along with having no reliable health care, the poor are increasingly less likely to live long enough to enjoy the good life, a good life whose promise is a fantasy that justifies so much exploitation? How do we think about labor- and consumer-related subjectivities in the same moment since one cannot talk about scandals of the appetite—food, sex, smoking, shopping, and drinking—merely as sites of moral approbation? Social policy in the domain of self-medication must look at the pressures of the workday, the debt cycle, consumer practice, and fantasy. Finally, what does it mean that African Americans and Latino/as are especially bearing this bodily burden along with the symbolic negativity long attached to it, so much so that one physician, a member of the Black Women's Health

Network, observes that the "most lethal weapon" against African American people in the contemporary United States is the fork?[10]

In short, the bodies of U.S. waged workers will be more fatigued, be in more pain, be less capable of ordinary breathing and working, and die earlier than the bodies of higher income workers, who are also getting fatter, but at a slower rate, and with relatively more opportunity for exercise.[11] Apart from working-class and subproletarian white women, who are more successful in mobilizing bourgeois beauty norms for economic success in the service sector, the overweight and obese poor will find it harder to get and keep jobs, remain healthy, and afford health care for the ensuing diseases.[12] They will become progressively more sedentary not just from the increasing passivity of more sedentary kinds of service work, not just from working more jobs more unevenly, not just because of television, and not just because there are fewer and fewer public spaces in which it is safe and pleasurable to walk, but because it is harder to move, period. They will live the decay of their organs and bodies more explicitly, more painfully, and more overwhelmingly than ever before, and it has become statistically clear that between stress and comorbidity they will die at ages younger than their grandparents and parents.[13] As one African American essayist describes the ongoing familial and cultural lure of the four American food groups—sugar, fat, salt, and caffeine—slow death affords what there is left of the good life for the vast majority of American workers.[14]

The epidemiological and political analysis I've focused on here does not much think about what people do when they are eating. I want to close in a different register, brainstorming a bit about what eating is in light of the daily life pressures and environments I've been describing. This redescription is not just a pleasure of mine, but an attempt to get a clearer sense of why it is so hard to intervene in the areas of appetites and pleasures without doing a lot of damage to the population most in crisis.

My focus here is on seeing eating as a kind of self-medication, but then rethinking what self-medication is. Marianne Valverde argues that self-medication isn't merely a weakness of those with diseases of the will.[15] It is often an understandable response to feeling overwhelmed, raw, a misfit. It is also often part of being in a community organized through promises of comfort in a generalized environment of belonging that might be personal (if one is a "regular" somewhere) or anonymous (if one is merely somewhere). Spreading out in these locations can be a temporal, episodic thing, and yet it extends being in the world undramatically.[16] The conviviality of consumption from this perspective marks duration: a different definition of "slow food," a concept and a movement that advocates for a way to counter the speeds with which capitalist activity destroys its environments at the same time as it makes living possible.[17]

After all, food is one of the few spaces of controllable, reliable pleasure that people have. Additionally, unlike alcohol or other drugs, food is necessary to existence, part of care of the self, the reproduction of life. How to articulate those urgencies of necessity and pleasure within structural conditions of existence that militate against the flourishing of workers and consumers? The forms of pleasure-spreading I've just been describing are also folded into the activity of doing what's necessary to lubricate the body's movement through capitalized time's shortened circuit—not only speed-up at work but also the specific contexts where making a life involves getting through the day, the week, and the month. Time organized by the near future of the payment of bills and the management of children coexists with the well-being a meal can provide. And although one might imagine that the knowledge of unhealthiness would make parents force themselves and their children into a different food regime, ethnographies of working-class families suggest that economic threats to the family's continuity and the parents' sense of well-being tend to produce households in which food is one of the few stress relievers and one of the few sites of clear continuity between children and parents.[18] Moreover, in scenes of economic struggle kids take on parental stress and seek comfort where the parents do as well, even as they cultivate small differences between adult and children's styles. The complexity of maintaining dependency identifications is simplified, in a sense, in filial relations of eating that function as a scene for the production of happiness in the terms of repeatable pleasure, if not health.

This is the material context for so many: working life exhausts practical sovereignty, the exercise of the will in the scene of the contingencies of survival. At the same time that one builds a life, the pressures of its reproduction can be experienced as exhausting. Eating is a form of ballast against wearing out, but it is also a counter-dissipation. Just like other forms of small pleasure, it can produce an experience of self-abeyance, of floating sideways. In this view, it's not synonymous with agency in the tactical or effectual senses dedicated to self-negation or self-extension, but self-suspension. I am not trying to replace a notion of cognitive will with a notion of involuntary or unconscious activity. In the model I am articulating, both the body and "a life" are not only projects, but also sites of episodic intermission from personality, ways of inhabiting agency differently in small vacations from the will itself, which is so often spent from the pressures of coordinating one's pacing with the pace of the working day, including times of preparation and recovery from this workday. Its pleasures can be seen as interrupting the liberal and capitalist subject called to consciousness, intentionality, and effective will. Self-interruption and the will to survive are not opposites, of course: that is my point. But the other point is that in this scene—where mental and physical health might actually be conflicting aims—the activity of riding a different wave of spreading out or shifting in the everyday also reveals confusions about what it means to have a life. Is it to have health? To love, to have been loved? Is it to achieve a state or a sense of worked-toward enjoyment? Is having a life the process one gets resigned to, after dreaming of the good life, or not even dreaming? Or is "life" as the scene of reliable pleasures located largely in those experiences of coasting, with all that's implied in that phrase, the shifting, sensual space between pleasure and numbness?

Whatever we do to make a life is, therefore, not usually a project of making oneself or the world *better*, but instead involves attention to making a less bad experience: a reprieve. While this domain of acts is not all unconscious—eating involves many kinds of self-understanding, especially in a culture of shaming and self-consciousness around the moral mirror choosing pleasures so often provides—it is often consciously and unconsciously not about imagining the long haul. The structural position of subaltern lives intensifies this foreshortening of consciousness and fantasy. Under a regime of crisis ordinariness, life feels truncated, more like doggy paddling than swimming out to a magnificent horizon in which all acts accumulate into an impact that can be enjoyed. The agency of eating can make interruptive episodes happen in which suspending the desire to be building toward the good life in rational ways involves cultivating a feeling of well-being that spreads out for a moment, not as a projection toward a future. Paradoxically, of course, at least during this phase of capital, there is less of a future when one eats without an orientation toward it.

What does all this say about the cruel and unusual nourishment of everyday life in the United States? For reasons beyond the sovereign fantasy, maybe the appetitive person is a little like the body politic. Both look constantly for reasons not to give up; both experience cycles of feeling detached, depressed, hopeful, and euphoric; both sense a threat of lost resilience altogether. Still, once in awhile, an episode interrupts the cycle. In these episodes, we throw our lot in with this ideology, that candidate, this snack, that meal in the hope that finally a durable kind of life will arrive where there are more pleasures than defeats. Let's call it the life drive: whatever else they are, the gestures that create "self-medicating" or lightening spaces in time exhibit fidelity to mental health, to happiness. They refuse the productive system's insistence that you wear yourself out in order to live.

Mainly people do not live very well in these spaces. For ordinary workers, this attrition of life or pacing of death where the everyday evolves within the complex processes of globalization, law, and state regulation is an old story in a new era.[19] The privileged have slightly more resources for resisting these modes of exhaustion, using their stretched time to eat well, exercise, vacation, and sleep. But hardly. For most, the overwhelming present is less well symbolized by vitalizing images of sustainable life, less guaranteed than ever by the glorious promise of bodily longevity and social security, than it is expressed in regimes of exhausted practical sovereignty, distracted agency, and, sometimes, counter-absorption in episodic refreshment—in sex, in spacing out, in food that is not for thought.

NOTES

1. David Harvey, "The Body as Accumulation Strategy," in *Spaces of Hope* (Berkeley: University of California Press, 2000), 97–116.

2. Available in World Health Organization documents as early as 1998, and registering typical anxiety about the joke-and-threat status of obesity in public sphere Western rhetoric about it, "globesity" is now in wide circulation in medical and commercial venues. See, for example, George Anderson, "Buzzwords *du Jour*: Prosumers, Metrosexuals, Globesity," *Retail Wire*, September 26, 2003, http://retailwire.com/Discussions/Sngl_Discussion.cfm/9272; Donna Eberwine, "Globesity: The Crisis of Growing Proportions," *Perspectives in Health Magazine: The Magazine of the Pan American Health Organization* 7, no. 3 (2002), http://www.paho.org/English/DPI/Number15_article2_5.htm; Stuart Blackman, "The Enormity of Obesity," The Scientist 18, no. 10 (May 24, 2004), http://the-scientist.com/yr2004/may/feature_040524.html; and multiple articles in *JAMA* and other medical journals. For a recent academic deployment of the term, see Don Kulick and Anne Meneley, "Introduction," in *Fat: The Anthropology of an Obsession* (New York: Jeremy P. Tarcher/Penguin, 2004).

3. The bill was introduced and passed in the House of Representatives in March 2004; the Senate version of the hamburger bill passed on October 19, 2005. See *Personal Responsibility in Food Consumption Act of 2005*, 109th Cong., 1st sess., H.R. 554, http://thomas.loc.gov/cgi-bin/query/D?c109:3:./temp/~c109WGW4wP::. For a legal/cultural reading of this event, see Dalia Lithwick, "My Big Fattening Greek Salad: Are French Fries the New Marlboros?" *Slate*, August 14, 2003, http://www.slate.com/id/2086970/.

4. See Laurie Tarkan, "Bananas, Maybe. Peas and Kale? Dream On," *New York Times*, June 21, 2005, http://www.nytimes.com/2005/06/21/health/nutrition/21pick.html?ex=1130126400&en=e8330837b26798f1&ei=5070; Melanie Warner, "California Wants to Serve a Warning with Fries," *New York Times*, September 21, 2005, http://www.nytimes.com/2005/09/21/business/21chips.html; Roni Rabin, "Study or No, Fries are Still Bad News," *Newsday*, September 20, 2005, http://www.newsday.com/news/columnists/

ny-hsroni204433178sep20,0,7848310.column?coll=ny-health-columnists. See also the response from business, for example, *Investors Business Daily*, "California's Low-Fact Diet," October 13, 2005.

5. Eric Oliver, Paul Campos, and Richard Klein, for instance, fight the "cold facts" of the obesity epidemic with their own cold facts, many of which are taken from "fat activists" who proffer their own anti-normative analyses of what should constitute definitions of health and sickness. Speaking a debunking language in the register of scandal to drown out the register of crisis, they do not write with a nuanced understanding of their participation in the discursive, and always processual, historical construction of disease.

6. Roland Sturm, "Increases in Clinically Severe Obesity in the United States, 1986–2000," *Archives of Internal Medicine* 163.18 (October 13, 2003): 2146–48. This fact was reported on throughout the United States. See, for example, the Associated Press report, "Fat Americans Getting Fatter," *CNN*, October 14, 2003. The United Kingdom is comparably described. See http://www.esrcsocietytoday.ac.uk/ESRCInfoCentre/facts/index55.as px?ComponentId=12741&SourcePageId=6970. The increase is also being tracked among adolescents. See Richard A. Miech, Shiriki K. Kumanyika, Nicolas Stettler, Bruce G. Link, Jo C. Phelan, and Virginia W. Chang, "Trends in the Association of Poverty With Overweight Among US Adolescents, 1971–2004,"
JAMA: Journal of the American Medical Association 295, no. 20 (May 24/31, 2006): 2385–93.

7. Gary Gardner and Brian Halweil, "Underfed and Overfed: The Global Epidemic of Malnutrition," *Worldwatch*, March 1, 2000, http://www.worldwatch.org/node/840. The pandemic nature of unhealthy overweight is registered in countless places. See research summaries in: Sue Y. S. Kimm and Eva Obarzanek, "Childhood Obesity: A New Pandemic of the New Millennium," *Pediatrics* 110, no. 5 (November 2002): 1003–7; Barry M. Popkin, "Using Research on the Obesity Pandemic as a Guide to a Unified Vision of Nutrition," *Public Health Nutrition* 8, no. 1 (September 2005): 724–29(6); A.R.P. Walker, "The Obesity Pandemic. Is It Beyond Control?" *Journal of the Royal Society for the Promotion of Health* 123, no. 3 (September 2003): 150–51. While increasing homogeneity of food distribution in global urban and suburban contexts has made unhealthy overweight a global medical concern, at the same time the norms of what constitutes evidence of bodily thriving remain resolutely local. See Natalie Angier, "Who Is Fat? It Depends on Culture," *New York Times*, November 7, 2000, http://www.nytimes.com/2000/11/07/science/who-is-fat-it-depends-on-culture.html.

8. A huge literature exists on the translocal impact of U.S. food policy and neoliberal market practices (often called "reforms") on global food production. A good general introduction to the field is Tim Lang and Michael Heasman, *Food Wars: The Global Battle for Minds, Mouths, and Markets* (London: Earthscan, 2004). But for a sense of the texture of the debates, it is most instructive to track the series of reports on food production politics, policies, and consequences at the World Trade Organization and World Social Forum meetings. You can do this at alternet.org and opendemocracy.org.

9. Of course, sensible people have argued that obesity and overweight are forms of resistance to the hegemony of the productive/bourgeois body as well as to white class-aspirational beauty culture. My counterargument is that while many forms of ordinary behavior can be phrased in terms of blockage, defense, or aggression, people are more vague and incoherent than this characterization would suggest. There is, in any case, a difference between eating and being fat, and both kinds of activity can be non-commu-

nicative gestures or ways of detaching from, or merely interrupting, a moment. Tracking how people shift within different modes of their own agency requires quite a different imaginary with regard to what it means to do something than is expressed in the transformative fantasy that saturates the concepts of resistance and protest. The scene of this chapter—the obesity epidemic and contexts for thinking about what eating does—is an obstacle to our appetite for drama. So, maybe, sometimes resistance is being acted out in these domains—but mainly not.

10. Dr. Patricia Davidson, "Opening and Welcome," "Unequal Burden," and "Access to Care," National Black Women's Health conference, April 11, 2003, *http://docs. google.com/gview?a=v&q=cache%3AaAKk9qBo53AJ%3Awww.kaisernetwork.org%2Fhealth_ cast%2Fuploaded_files%2Fo41103_nbwhp_morning.pdf+patricia+davidson+unequal+burden +access+to+care&hl=en&gl=us&pli=1.*

11. See Kenneth F. Adams, Arthur Schatzkin, Tamara B. Harris, Victor Kipnis, Traci Mouw, Rachel Ballard-Barbash, Albert Hollenbeck, and Michael F. Leitzmann, "Overweight, Obesity, and Mortality in a Large Prospective Cohort of Persons 50 to 71 Years Old," *New England Journal of Medicine* 355, no. 8 (August 24, 2006): 763–78.

12. For a variety of comparisons between women's eating and mobility patterns, see Jeffery Sobal and Albert J. Stunkard, "Socioeconomic Status and Obesity: A Review of the Literature," *Psychological Bulletin* 105, no. 2 (March 1989): 260–75; Meg Lovejoy, "Disturbances in the Social Body: Differences in Body Image and Eating Problems Among African American and White Women," *Gender and Society* 15, no. 2 (April 2001): 239–61. See also See Virginia W. Chang, "U.S. Obesity, Weight Gain, and Socioeconomic Status," *CHERP Policy Brief* 3, no. 1 (2005); Virginia W. Chang and Diane Lauderdale, "Income Disparities in Body Mass Index and Obesity in the United States, 1971–2002," *Archives of Internal Medicine* 165, no. 18 (October 10, 2005): 2122–28; and Virginia W. Chang and Nicholas A. Christakis, "Income Inequality and Weight Status in US Metropolitan Areas," *Social Science and Medicine* 61, no. 1 (July 2005): 83–96.

Chang's work alone demonstrates the lability of contemporary accounts of the class and racial indicators of overweightness and obesity. In "U.S. Obesity, Weight Gain, and Socioeconomic Status," she argues that poverty-related obesity presents a variety of significant healthcare challenges in the United States, while claiming that the rate of increase in obesity currently varies significantly across class and locale and that middle-class nonwhites are increasing their degree of overweightness faster than the poor. In "Income Inequalities," though, she and her co-author note that varying degrees of economic inequality in different metropolitan areas does not much affect individuals' risk of obesity, except for white women who continue to use weight status as a means of class mobility. The implication of the latter article is that income inequality in the United States does not *create* weight-related unhealth, but the implication of "Income Disparities" is that there is nonetheless a *high correlation* between individual income and unhealthy weight because the poor are indeed more likely to be significantly overweight than everyone else. This tension between causality and correlation is what creates much of the polemical and methodological debate over whether weight-related unhealth in the United States presents an epidemic, a problem, or even an interesting phenomenon.

13. For a useful summary of the current literature, see Debra J. Brown, "Everyday Life for Black American Adults: Stress, Emotions, and Blood Pressure," *Western Journal of Nursing Research* 26, no. 5 (August 2004): 499–514. While the specter of shorter life has

been tracked in the medical and popular press for a while, the clearest current epidemiological representation of this phenomenon is S. Jay Olshansky, Douglas J. Passaro, Ronald C. Hershow, Jennifer Layden, Bruce A. Carnes, Jacob Brody, Leonard Hayflick, Robert N. Butler, David B. Allison, and David S. Ludwig, "A Potential Decline in Life Expectancy in the United States in the 21st Century," *New England Journal of Medicine* 352, no. 11 (March 17, 2005): 1138–45. The popular debate continues. Just after the publication of Rob Stein, "Obesity May Stall Trend of Increasing Longevity," *Washington Post*, March 17, 2005, a counterargument was staged in *Scientific American*. See W. Wayt Gibbs, "Obesity: An Overblown Epidemic?" *Scientific American*, May 23, 2005, http://www.scientificamerican.com/article.cfm?id=obesity-an-overblown-epid.

14. Dyann Logwood, "Food for Our Souls," in *Body Outlaws: Young Women Write About Body Image & Identity*, ed. Ophira Edut (Seattle: Seal Press, 2000), 98.

15. See Marianne Valverde, *Diseases of the Will: Alcohol and the Dilemmas of Freedom* (New York: Cambridge University Press, 1998).

16. In using eating in excess of caloric requirements for the reproduction of life as a way to think about lateral agency and some contexts of its materialization, I am refuting the kinds of misconstrual that characterize the subject of appetites (e.g., "people") as always fully present to their motives, desires, feelings, and experiences, or as even desiring to be. For a brilliant performance of this error which goes through all the actuarial and historical material one could want while insisting on a hypercognitive historical actor presently obsessed with eating and fat, see Richard Klein, *Eat Fat* (New York: Pantheon, 1996). For a beautifully written but even more self-contradictory performance of this perspective, see Elspeth Probyn, "Eating Sex," in *Carnal Appetites: Foodsexidentities* (London: Routledge, 2000), 59–77. Adapting Deleuze and Guattari's articulation of the sexual and the alimentary, Probyn argues paradoxically that eating is at once a performative part of the becoming central to the ongoing undoing of the subject in assemblages of processual sensual activity *and* that the appetitive is nonetheless exemplary as a grounding site of self-discovery, self-confirmation, identity, and ethics.

17. The "slow food" movement that emerged in Europe in the 1990s responds to many of the same environmental factors that this chapter details. Along with its critique of neoliberal agricultural policies, it translates the impulsive improvisation around recalibrating the pacing of the day into a collective program for deliberative being in the world in a way opposed to the immediatist, productive one of anxious capital. For a terrific analysis of the phenomenon, see Alison Leitch, "Slow Food and the Politics of Pork Fat: Italian Food and European Identity," *Ethnos* 68, no. 4 (December 2003): 437–62.

18. See Lillian B. Rubin, *Worlds of Pain: Life in the Working-Class Family* (New York: Basic Books, 1977), and Jody Heymann, *Forgotten Families: Ending the Growing Crisis Confronting Children and Working Parents in the Global Economy* (New York: Oxford University Press, 2006).

19. See, for example, Mike Davis's stunning *Late Victorian Holocausts: El Niño Famines and the Making of the Third World* (New York: Verso, 2001).

4

Against Global Health?

Arbitrating Science, Non-Science, and
Nonsense through Health[1]

VINCANNE ADAMS

Early in the wake of the millennium, the idea of global health began to take hold in the world of international development aid. By 2006, programs in "International Health" throughout the United States began to rename themselves and create subsidiary programs in "Global Health." The University of California, San Francisco graduated the first class of master's degree students in Global Health Sciences in 2009. "Global Health," as distinguished from "International Health," was meant to encompass the interconnectedness of all countries (rich or poor, North or South) in a mission to create health on a global scale. In so doing, it provided a salvo for postcolonial critiques of unidirectional and binary models of international aid. Questions about what exactly the shift to "global health" has entailed, however, have yet to be fully mapped and sufficiently answered.[2] In what follows, I explore the shift to global health as more than a component of globalization, more than a corrective to postcolonial bilateralism. In this chapter, I offer a critical exploration of the processes by which the notion of "health" in Global Health Sciences holds a tyrannical relationship to problems within the actual practices of global health.

The notion of "health" as something that can only be accomplished through scientific rigor simultaneously emerges alongside scientific practices that sometimes conceal and arbitrate social practices of inequality and erasure, all the while claiming to "fix" certain problems. Health can sometimes become a mechanism of politics by embedding itself in the world of science, and by distinguishing itself from its comparative counterparts: non-science and nonsense. This process of epistemological boundary-making is accomplished through social relationships crossing several disciplines, histories, and terrains of intention. I begin the story with an encounter between doctors, scientists, and social scientists.

Global Health

In 2007, a group of physicians and global health researchers at my university (University of California, San Francisco) planned a workshop on "Global Health Diplomacy," a field that was to explore the politics of intervention in the emerging assemblages of "Global Health Science."[3] At one point, I raised a question about the ways in which our workshop would discuss problems of health and politics. An anthropological perspective, I offered, would consider a variety of analytical frames: "biopower," "biological citizenship," "therapeutic citizenship." These were the new technologies of governance in a postcolonial world. Health interventions, I noted, not only addressed disease and morbidity, but in some sense also obligated recipients to become model subjects, swiftly replacing old regimes of governance in organizing civil society.[4] AIDS prevention programs, for example, teach subjects how to have and not have sex, how to negotiate marital relations, how to become "outreach workers" in prevention programs. These programs were not just aimed at health, but at new ways of being citizens in an AIDS-filled community and thus were centrally about the political.

One of my physician colleagues, however, bristled at the mention of these notions. "Biowhat? That seems overly theoretical to me. Health and politics," he said, "simply means using political negotiations to achieve health goals." He suggested that we focus on things like the World Health Organization Framework Convention on Tobacco Control, the Oslo Accords, and the building of CDC branches in China. Social analyses, even those that were about politics, were too vague and unscientific for use, according to him. Health was not a rubric for analyzing modern relations of power enacted through public interventions. Rather, health was the goal of interventions, and politics was simply a tool for getting there.

In the end, our workshop focused on global treaties rather than on the micropolitics of development citizenship, but the deliberations raised a number of questions about what sorts of knowledge and what sorts of scientific framing "count" in health contexts, and also how these framings count in comparison to one another in relation to interventions that claim to have health as their explicit goal. The experience raised my interest in tracing the shift from "international health" to "Global Health Sciences" in order to explore how the commitment to health—the singular goal of global health programs—often becomes the means by which such programs authorize subtle shifts between epistemological frames: between science, non-science, and nonsense. In these shifts, it becomes possible to see how health some-times works to conceal and erase some truths while foregrounding others, even when some of these truths might actually be seen as critical to staying or being well.

Science and Non-Science:
From Colonial to Postcolonial International Health

International health emerged as a new field of research and intervention in the post–World War II period, as decolonization was partnered with the cre-ation of multinational, multilateral aid organizations aimed at shifting finan-cial and infrastructural resources from the former colonizing to the newly decolonized world.[5] International Health, of course, was actually a new name for programs that borrowed from and built upon the epistemic frameworks from previous medical programs that had worked in tandem with colonial-ism.[6] Colonial medicine had long been practiced as a tool for improving the health of natives, saving them (spiritually and physically) from their own medical ignorance, and ensuring a stable labor force.[7]

From the perspective of international public health, the "sciences" of health have thus always had global contours. Colonial and missionary medi-cine from the nineteenth century onward made use of biological sciences to frame, audit, and advance colonial activities[8] as well as to advance science at home by way of the colonial experience.[9] In these iterations, scientific approaches to disease and disease prevention and control were deployed as population-level concerns embedded in the rubrics of tropical medicine, hygiene, pathology, and evolution, to name a few. Science, in this context, was eventually tied to an empirical world of viruses, bacteria, and parasites that exacted a toll and became visible through patients, populations, and physicians.

To obtain health at the individual or population level, colonial medicine advocated public health measures to treat or immunize against infectious dis-eases and to teach the natives how to avoid contracting these diseases in the first place through behavioral change. Scientific studies provided the guide-lines that enabled health to be achieved in these programs. In most cases, the doctors involved were also the scientists, logging records of infection, treatment successes, and in some cases studying the pathology of diseases. Theories of contagion and the biology and ecology of things like hookworm, sleeping sickness, yaws, malaria, and tuberculosis formed the world of "sci-entific medicine" in this era. The focus of such studies was on developing strategies to combat deadly epidemics and the chronic lassitude that resulted from the endemic forms of these infectious and parasitic agents. The colonial tropics were a virtual smorgasbord for health scientists that held dual investments in understanding the science of pathogens and in developing effective treatment regimes.

Medical science in this era was driven by a clinical imperative that drew from and focused on the health needs of both native and colonial. Science in this context may have used microscopes, bacterial samples, and reagents, but the foundational ground for its inquiries was always health as seen in real patients with real diseases. This could be contrasted with later efforts to pursue "science" as an end in and of itself through colonial or postcolonial medicine. As we will see, this orientation changed significantly over the years, eventually giving rise to Global Health Sciences and leading to a shift from health to "science." This shift entailed management of the thorny problem of what would and should constitute "science" along the way.

International "health" in the colonial era positioned itself against, and in some way built its own sense of mission by positioning itself against, non-science—that is, traditional beliefs about spirits, witchcraft, demonic possessions, and a host of other "irrational" folk beliefs about the causes of illness and disease. Natives did things like provide enemas for infant diarrhea, which exacerbated dehydration and speeded death. They believed that eating from the clean hands of a low caste person was more dangerous than eating from the bacteria-filled hands of a person of high caste.[10] They used herbal concoctions and ritual cures for what could, in the scientific mind, only be effectively treated with antibiotics.[11] Contrasted with "science," traditional beliefs were not merely non-scientific in the colonial medical mind-set; they seemed to be "nonsense" as empirical explanations of medical facts. Effective interventions carried the authority of science behind them, and non-science was not only useless to these interventions but actually dangerous. Natives who treated their children's acute respiratory infections with shamanic exorcisms were not just ignorant. They revealed a more dangerous scourge—aberrant thought.[12] Colonial-era anthropologists, poised to rectify at least the ethnocentrism of colonialism, inventoried these beliefs for their logic, rationality, and symbolic effectiveness, but they did not call them "scientific."[13]

These contrary categories of medical logic—one considered scientific and the other not—formed a continuous presence through decolonization and the rise of international health.[14] The sciences of twentieth-century public health, upon which international health was built as a distinct field of scholarship and intervention in the postcolonial context, have changed. Epidemiology, and pathology, ecology, and economics (rather than evolution) were used throughout the latter half of the twentieth century and continue to be used to promote health internationally. These health sciences took and continue to take practical and clinical form in programs for reproductive health and contraception, immunization, cold-chain storage, oral rehydration, the distribution of mosquito nets, access to safe drinking water, the promotion of safe sex, and HIV prevention, to name a few.[15] The clinically driven health sciences have made use of prior colonial conceptualizations of the bases for health and disease, even as they have moved away from being articulated through overtly colonial regimes.

International health programs that emerged in the postwar, postcolonial era still distinguish between scientific and other kinds of "traditional" medical knowledge, and in many ways the rubric of health itself has authorized a continuous need for distinguishing between these kinds of knowledge. Interventions are promoted based on the assumption that if morbidity's causes can be known scientifically, they can be prevented and even eradicated with the proper medical interventions. If villagers continue to see disease in a non-scientific, nonsensical way—that is, as a result of spirit attack, evil eye, loss of soul—then health will never be achieved. Ignorance is the real cause of disease—ignorance of truths that arrive via international health programs, some of which must anticipate their emergent targets even before they arrive.[16] In these international health programs, the notion that health is only possible if pursued as a scientific goal is seldom questioned.

Postcolonial international health development has formed a nexus that intertwines health with science and within which the solution to all ills—from poverty to political repression—is frequently tied directly to health. For example, reproductive health and child survival are tied to population reduction and economic prosperity; child nutrition programs are tied to small business loans for mothers; infrastructural aid is rationalized as a key to healthy families. Integrated health development, starting in the late 1970s, positioned health at the center of economic, infrastructural, and educational development constellations, making it clear that at the core of successful development was not simply a high national GNP but a low threshold of morbidity overall and reduced mortality (especially for under-five-year-olds). Here too, the sciences of economy and ecology brought empirical understandings of the links between health, disease, and the survival of nation-states to the forefront, making the health/science nexus more visible than ever.

Even in the postwar era, however, scientific facts about health and its attainment continued to rely on the assumption that scientific knowledge is constitutively different from traditional belief, despite anthropological efforts to trouble this relationship.[17] In postcolonial health development endeavors, anthropological contributions to international health have grown in importance and in the scope of their contribution.[18] Placed somewhere in the middle of the continuum between the "nonsense" of traditional beliefs and the "science" of biomedical claims, ethnographic research is usually treated as a kind of "soft science" in service to the "hard." Anthropologists study the social and cultural beliefs and behaviors that explain things like why target populations use traditional methods of healing (even though they are dangerous from a Western medical perspective); why villagers refuse appropriate, scientifically based treatments (despite their effectiveness); and why these people insist on treating health as something that can only be achieved within the context of larger social relationships and cultural arrangements.[19]

In many of these studies, the logic of traditional health behaviors is embedded in local understandings of larger sociopolitical inequities. Brazilian mothers might choose to selectively neglect infants who appear sickly and weak because, under conditions of socioeconomic scarcity, they know only the babies who are born with the ability to struggle for life will survive.[20] Haitian victims of AIDS/SIDA may blame their disease on sorcery because, from their perspective, the disease is actually sent by envious and corrupt outsiders. But these sociopolitical renderings of the traditional causes of disease often still have to pass through the sieve of scientific explanation. Starvation, dehydration, malnutrition, and HIV infection are comprehensible as primarily biological processes that can be undone and prevented with the right interventions. The social scientist calls for political and social reforms to end inequality, and the health developer calls for health reforms that teach mothers not to neglect their children. Sometimes, these two objectives are merged.

In any case, critical anthropological insights brought to bear on international health offer a subtle displacement of the boundary between science and non-science in the new era of international health, making traditional behaviors sensible if still not healthful and making their own insights stand up as comparable to science. Political causes of disease are as important as microbial ones,[21] but social science is still not "science" in the same way as that word is used in the term "health sciences." In the end, the tight nexus joining health to science continues to define the nature and direction of interventions within international health, sometimes making it seem that social science insights are not tied directly to health itself.

This framing of the ongoing dichotomy between science and non-science underpins and explains the reaction of my physician colleague who felt that social theory overly complicated and in some sense missed the real target of intervention: health. In his view, anthropological analysis can provide interesting understandings of the logics of non-science, but these logics are still not scientifically sensible or practical from the perspective of interventionist medicine. The reaction recalls a familiar refrain between medicine and medical anthropology, one that hinges on a temporal framing of value: policy aimed at effecting health behaviors is useful in ways that studies of the effects of health intervention policies cannot be. Social science analytics are not useful when they carry no obvious front-end impact for intervention—that is, when they are not focused on ways of actually bringing health into being. To point out that political or social interventions are needed is not, for the traditional health development expert, a novel idea; it is impractical, if not useless. Social science, in most international health circles, becomes a kind of non-science whose relevance can only be justified by its ability to advance real, scientifically based interventions, which in turn are based on the foregrounding of health above all other goals. Like traditional beliefs, social science insights are not nonsense, but they are categorically not "science" in the way that medicine is because they displace the focus from health to things like social inequality, political injustice, and cultural discrimination. These things are just too large and amorphous to tackle if health is the goal.[22] Much of this has changed, however, with the emergence of "global health sciences."

Global Health Sciences

Today, global health sciences bring to international public health a new kind of "science" in the form of pharmaceutical research, clinical drug testing, and laboratory concerns (such as how to collect blood samples and how to store them in resource-poor settings, how to train scientists from local communities, how to create supply chains for laboratory equipment and materials). That is, conventional approaches to the field and the work of international health have been joined by a growing interest in melding bench and laboratory sciences and pharmaceutical research with the old familiar terrain of advancing "Health for all," the WHO millennial goal from the late 1980s. The shift has entailed, I would argue, a move away from the focus on "health/science" to a focus on "science," or at least a focus on science as separable from health both strategically and selectively.

The Global Health Sciences degree at UCSF was created in part to aid and create community among bench scientists who were suddenly globalizing. New issues of funding, institutional review boards, collaborations with host countries, and patenting were put on the table. Laboratory researchers working on developing HIV antiretrovirals in Uganda, on the blood genetics of diabetes in the Caribbean, on stem cell procurement in Taiwan, or on the clinical testing of new drugs in naïve populations outside the United States were brought together with international health experts who formerly worked for USAID, the WHO, and the CDC. Within these rubrics, the guiding principle of health enabled two sides of the world of health sciences to begin talking in new ways. The clinical orientation of public health experts and doctors familiar with international health were brought face to face with biochemists, virologists, and molecular biologists who wanted to extend their laboratories beyond the edges of their own nations and populations. The natural alliance between these fields, already in place within medical schools in the large universities of the developed world, has become a new sort of exploration for those working abroad. Health is what unites them but, as I would say, science is what divides them.

Clinical physicians and public health advocates were presented with new challenges as UCSF pushed to franchise research laboratories in disparate regions of the world, a move they presented as the next wave of "health development." There were positive ways of reading this from a public health perspective. Building scientific communities of research in places like Kinshasa would stem the "brain drain" of qualified local physicians and researchers. The development of private-public partnerships in research science, it was argued, would create new kinds of sustainability for health infrastructure in under-resourced nations. In the most optimistic circles, one heard talk of the benefits of globalized clinical trials that would provide new medical resources to populations that had previously been unable to obtain them. That is, when it came to accounting for the positive outcomes of a global health science, health was then and is now foregrounded as the benefit and reward of such endeavors and mergers.

The mergers formed in Global Health Sciences have, however, generated awkward and troubling outcomes. Adriana Petryna, Joao Biehl, Arthur Kleinman, Andrew Lakoff, Ian Whitmarsh and others have offered cautionary insights about these new alliances, including the ways in which contract research organization-based pharmaceutical trials displace the objectives of public health, making it difficult for many of the poor in these regional locations to obtain health care except by enrolling in clinical trials. They have shown that pharmaceutical priorities in global health sciences can lead to an effacing of a whole range of local health problems because certain diseases and maladies have more pharmaceutical research potential.[23] Furthermore, drug testing produces ethical eddies into which the most vulnerable are lured.[24] They note that research incentives within science have a way of imposing racial and social inequalities on study populations as a result of the prioritizing of statistical- and evidence-based imperatives over health concerns.[25] In some measure, it is the prioritizing of pharmaceutical consumption and its research agenda over the prioritizing of health that leads to these problems, and yet, it is important to recall that there is still a way in which global health sciences, which is also undertaken in the name of health, might be cause for another kind of concern.

Amidst the growing industries of global health, I would point to a nested and somewhat less discussed piece of the trouble that arrives with the marriage of pharmaceutical and bench sciences with international health work. As pharmaceutical and clinical research take up more and more space in the world of public health, the notion of what is "scientific" and, alongside this, the notion of what is "healthy" have shifted. Rubrics of science that circulate in the world of the laboratory take on a type of empirical tyranny in comparison to other practices in medicine. Randomization, the use of controls, double blinds, power calculations, and the idea of using only statistically valid results begin to circulate as the measures of efficacy that must be met in global health efforts. Public health programs seem "non-scientific" in view of the more rigorous versions of science that come to the global health table. Along with this, notions of health are less and less visible at the level of the individual or the population, but more visible at the level of the repaired organ, the CD4 count, and the fact that more subjects consider themselves eligible for operations.[26]

A good example of the ways that notions of health have shifted with the rise of global health sciences comes from my research into Tibetan doctors who are rapidly modernizing their research techniques to meet international randomized clinical trial standards. One physician who works on liver diseases told me that he is trying to develop a research platform to show that Tibetan medicines are effective at improving liver function in cases of hepatitis, cirrhosis, and cancer. He attended a conference in Shanghai, he said, in which he was exposed to many of the biomedical research models for clinical studies. Then, he said:

One of the Western doctors from a Shanghai hospital gave an example of a case. He treated a patient and finally, in the end the patient was dead, but before he was dead, they checked his liver. The cancer got smaller, but the patient is dead. When they discussed the case, the cause of death, the doctors said "the treatment is successful," because the tumor was reduced, right? But at the meeting, many traditional Chinese doctors and many other doctors said that according to traditional Chinese and Tibetan medicine, this is not a success, because the patient is dead. Yes. It's true that you can reduce the tumors. But the patient is dead. So, how can you measure that as success? Western doctors said, in their discussion of the cause of death, they said, "Oh, this treatment is a success and this medicine is effective."[27]

The problem of defining where exactly health is located and how it should be measured is tied deeply to the ways in which notions of scientific research have been developed within global health sciences. The health of an organ is easily substituted for the survival of the patient in laboratory studies of the effectiveness of particular pharmaceuticals. The sense of shock on the part of this Tibetan doctor—that it is possible to consider the outcome of research a success even though a patient dies—requires embracing the notion that health itself could be located in a specific organ rather than in a whole person. In this logic, death itself was absorbed within the notion of health.

I learned this during my own research in the Tibetan Autonomous Region when our project to evaluate training in safe infant delivery techniques was scuttled by our funder, who told us, "Not enough women die in Tibet to get a good power calculation."[28] How would our program be able to find a control group? How could we ensure that our outcomes were statistically valid? Worst of all, our Ob-Gyn nurse-researcher insisted on transporting every village woman who was in delivery distress to the local hospital on each of our research visits, and we were told that this would "really mess up our numbers." We had to stop saving women like this. Here, the possibility of shifting the notion of health to that of a "good scientific outcome" for the sake of health down the road was unquestioned. Here, health moved along a temporal continuum; it demanded the sacrifice of some subjects for the sake of a potential future when large numbers of people might be made or kept healthy. It is a calculus of investment potential, not too unlike the one used by pharmaceutical companies to justify the erasure of one kind of empirical concern for another. The fact that some women might die without our help could be erased for the sake of obtaining more robust numbers that could tell us that more women could be saved in the future if we furthered our knowledge of the scientific "evidence base." The calculus of profit and loss here redefined what health might actually mean, once again making space for the "death" therein.

Problems of accountability are often packaged in terms of a contested territory of science. What counts as a valid measure of impact and what kind of science does this accounting require? The regimes of science arriving with globalized bench sciences ask for a different kind of rigor and data that make traditional programs in international health education, maternal and child health, poverty alleviation, and hygiene seem questionable. A new rhetoric of scientific accountability has made it seem incontestable to claim, as one article did in the *Journal of the American Medical Association* (*JAMA*), that "few global health interventions are evidence-based."[29] The idea of "evidence-based" medicine is itself contingent on both new kinds of calculi and new kinds of health.

Traditionally, reports about program effectiveness have been closely tied to the rhetorical styles of their funding organizations (whether Operation Smile or World Neighbors or the World Health Organization), with simple quantitative figures rather than reliable statistical analyses that show the impacts of programs or that these impacts can be attributed to the program rather than mere chance. In most cases, reports focused on cases that demonstrated to funders that the organization was doing good work—simple statistics about how many children were immunized; how many clinics opened; how many patients seen; the number of mothers who delivered safely. What previously stood for evidence of success were claims like the following from an earlier Gates Foundation endeavor: "The Global Alliance for Vaccines and Immunizations made 5-year commitments to 72 countries for $1.6 billion worth of support . . . leading to the vaccination of some 100 million children, sparing more than 1 million from premature death due to *Haemophilus influenzae* B, pertussis, hepatitis B, measles and other diseases."[30] Historically, in some health development circles, it was not even clear that reporting on measurable health impact was a priority. Efforts focused instead on what was still left to be done, justifying the need for more funding for further interventions.[31] In these circles, everyone knew that health, defined by these somewhat simple but rather clear measurables, was the primary goal, even if this health seemed perpetually unattainable.

The arrival of evidence-based medicine as a scientific platform in international health created a language within which to evaluate programs but also one which potential funders could use to ratchet up the surveillance that determined their support. "Evidence-based global health" is being pushed as the new way to do international health. This shift has made it more legitimate for international health research to be included in traditional, mainstream Western medical journals like *The Lancet* or *JAMA*. The new field of evidence-based global health, *JAMA* reports, "requires use of evidence from randomized controlled trials and other scientifically valid studies to evaluate global health interventions and to measure progress in improving global health." The authors of the same article suggest using "cluster trials, randomizing groups or communities."[32] This call has given rise to a new crop of articles in international public health and medical journals with subtitles like "a randomized, double-blind, controlled trial of [insert public health intervention and country name]." Tucked within these suggestions-cum-mandates in *JAMA*, we find new meanings of health, health outcomes, and health measures that can only become visible through the use of these technological and statistical calculations.

Perusing international health publications, one can find many exemplary cases of evidence-based global health. A study of "monthly antibiotic chemoprophylaxis and incidence of sexually transmitted infections and HIV-1 infection in Kenyan sex workers," for instance, was conducted as a randomized clinical trial.[33] Another article details a randomized comparative study of the effect of hand washing with soap on incidence of diarrhea among children in low-income neighborhoods in Karachi.[34] My favorite is the evidence-based randomized, controlled, and double-blind study conducted in Mexico that assessed the benefits of "a comprehensive program including fortified nutrition supplements for children and education, health care and cash transfers to [low-income] families."[35] The control group was given the same interventions delayed by one year. Not surprisingly, "investigators found that the intervention was associated with better growth in height and lower rates of anemia in low-income, rural infants and children."[36] In these cases, one finds a handy index for health—good statistics. But questions are seldom raised about whether or not the statistical evidence-making apparatuses are appropriate or inappropriate for the settings in which they are deployed.

The language of evidence-based science, randomization, controls, and robust statistical analysis is seen as a language that will provide new information that was not already "commonsense." Nevertheless, the shift in language has had a displacing effect, making public health efforts that do not produce these kinds of evidence seem "non-scientific" and therefore making not just their reports but the interventions themselves of questionable worth. The authors who praise these studies for taking a rigorous scientific approach seem shocked to learn that, in reviewing the literature on the benefits of providing nutritional supplements to low-income communities, there were only *two* randomized controlled trials on the growth monitoring of children.[37] Rather than generating a set of questions about what kinds of evidence should count in ascertaining the worthiness of nutritional supplement programs, publications like this tend to shift the terms of debate entirely and make it seem as if, without good scientific evidence, the interventions themselves are invalid. Common sense about these interventions is displaced by a narrow rhetoric of scientific truth that makes all evidence that is not packaged in these terms seem like nonsense because its validity cannot be established.

Within the new framework of evidence-based medicine, few contest or evaluate the ways in which basic notions of health are themselves being changed. For example, despite the fact that health outcomes are taken as given in most of this research (as if statistical results can unproblematically stand in for health itself), very few research efforts in global health sciences explore the ways in which different notions of health must be mobilized in order to obtain evidence that can be used in evidence-based medicine. Rather than simply study how many mothers use dietary supplements or come to nutrition programs, for instance, evidence-based studies require that some mothers not be given the supplements or nutrition programs and that measurable health status indicators be tied to the results. If you cannot come up with a valid health indicator (reduced incidence of diarrheal diseases, increased growth rates of children, etc.) then the intervention might be considered ill-conceived or not worth pursuing. These constraints change the notion of health that must be used to obtain funding and justify interventions, and they sometimes prevent good projects from being pursued at all.

In our planning for the Global Health Sciences degree at UCSF, clinical physicians found themselves marginalized in comparison to university laboratory researchers whose projects on the genetics of HIV and antiretrovirals in Uganda, or on malarial and TB pharmaceutics being tested in Mexico and the Caribbean. These researchers became the placeholders for building the Global Health Sciences department and they dictated the rubric for obtaining funding from donors like the Gates Foundation. In an environment where the agendas of bench science reigned, it was difficult for clinicians with years of experience in international health development to understand how to make comprehensive programs in health aid look methodologically "scientific."

International health programs designed to work with target country health ministries, for example, are often deployed as large-scale interventions that follow a general WHO or USAID mandate, rather than being tied to global discourse on the science of intervention. Health ministries often have priorities that conflict with those of the needs of scientific research. One researcher who was testing HIV prevention and contraception in several countries felt that it was much easier to work outside local health ministries. The health ministries' goals were often based on programs that would maximize care for the largest populations and prioritize those with the most need. In contrast, clinical researchers like this prefer to work in populations who had limited access to health resources, and they want to keep it this way since working in areas where there is access to multiple clinics that are not involved in the study means that patients may be able to obtain medicines that would confound the study results. In the world of international health aid, the idea that patients could obtain medicines from multiple sites (assuming they were reliable) would be read as a positive health outcome. For clinical researchers, however, such an outcome would be seen as a complicating factor in getting the sort of data needed for accurate studies. In clinical science, the notion of a positive health outcome has to be run through the sieve of randomization and control before it can be counted as positive or even valid.

Claims about what counts as a legitimate health problem are configured problematically in relation to the new arrival of pharmaceutical science. In our planning meetings, for example, health development experts found themselves wondering how and why programs that previously constituted important parts of health development work (education, sanitation, immunizations, and nutrition) might be able to find room at the table now that the focus had shifted to diseases for which clinical and laboratory research on specific pharmaceutical interventions had the lion's share of funding. We witnessed what Petryna noted, that infectious diseases that do not have bench science or pharmaceutical applications have a tendency to become invisible in global health research.

The Gates Foundation provides a good example of the shift toward this new kind of science. In 2002, the Foundation hired the former director of the National Cancer Institute, Richard Klausner, to run the foundation's global health program. One of his largest initiatives was "Grand Challenges in Global Health," which solicited proposals from a thousand scientists from all over the world to compete for funding to conduct research "that could lead to breakthroughs deemed most likely to improve health in poor countries."[38] They funded forty-three research projects that were mostly laboratory science–based research studies that linked developed and developing world interests. The program elicited the criticism that the foundation was simply replicating research that was already fundable by the National Institutes of Health in the United States. Klausner also promoted the Global HIV Vaccine Enterprise, partnering explicitly with the NIH. This program shifted resources from a focus on the delivery of vaccines and treatments to real people to a focus on laboratory research in immunology, drug development, and genetics, using populations for blood samples and as clinical trial subjects only. The merging of the bench with the field of global health sciences entails a re-engineering and refiguring of the notion of not only what constitutes a useful intervention but again, the very notion of health itself. Suddenly, health is something that can no longer be simply about the absence of illness or disease. Health is now tied invariably to the success or failure of research that advances our knowledge of immunology, genes, and randomization strategies. The "Grand Challenge of Global Health" is no longer simply about keeping patients alive; it is also about whether or not science can function stochastically and robustly in these contexts.

More generally, this transition is consistent with the growth in public-private partnerships (PPPs) in the world of global health, in which public partnering with pharmaceutical companies to re-invest in research on "neglected diseases" has resulted in an increased focus on drug and patent development. Research on questions of effective delivery and upon integrated development programs that ensure that eradication efforts are sustainable, equitable, population-based, as well as part of an overall program for improvement in living conditions and quality of life, becomes hard to manage within the frameworks of clinical trials.[39] Research priorities often trump the needs of patient care, even in the most ethical IRB-approved research studies.

Conclusion: Health as the Arbiter of Truth

In the maneuvering to claim ownership of "reliability" by using scientific techniques of accounting, health development clinicians try to keep the focus on intervention. As doctors, they are not necessarily scientists, even though their practices are scientifically derived. Most of the physicians I work with are activists; they are caregivers.[40] They are taught to treat disease and promote health, but they are not always prepared to do these things in the context of an evidence-based study. Turning the world of international health into a laboratory space for research can sometimes make some of them feel uncomfortable. I would suggest that this is in part because of the work that "health" is made to do as a signifier for more than just eliminating disease. It is made to do the work of generating scientific studies and producing evidence-based outcomes that don't always mesh well with the goals of patient care.

Globalized pharmaceutical research and the race to create the world of international health as a terrain for experimentation raise the question of what kind of science international health clinicians should align themselves with. As these clinicians are increasingly made to feel the need to be "scientific," they scale up and make rigorous experimental models for their work in ways that often take them further from the interventions they hope to deliver. Although many are enthusiastic about the new rigor in the field, some find it an infringement on their ability to provide adequate caregiving. Evidence-based requirements begin to look impractical and nonsensical when those planning interventions know that they cannot always establish controls in village-based healthcare efforts because randomization is nearly impossible to achieve within public health infrastructures and because doing double-blind studies is ethically impossible when it comes to programs in health education or immunization. Ironically, it is often this kind of fraught encounter that returns clinicians to discussions with the social scientists who, despite an apparent inability to leave behind jargon and theory, begin to look like more suitable partners in the effort to provide care than their colleagues sitting on laboratory benches. Although it is not always and certainly not uniformly true, in the new global health sciences social scientists sometimes appear concerned with outcomes and practical caregiving in ways that lab and bench scientists cannot because of their need for a specific kind of methodological rigor. In the social sciences, as in old-fashioned international health work, notions of health still authorize simple questions like, "is the patient getting better?" or "are more people able to get treatment?" These are questions that can be counted simply and without control trials. They also do not assume that, in the face of any interventions at all, chance can possibly account for these outcomes.

Despite its reputation as being "non-science" but not quite "nonsense," among my global health scientist colleagues, the social sciences offer something to the world of global health that may be useful. Recognizing the subtle shifts in the meanings of health that come with experimental research is perhaps just a starting point for a larger inquiry, but one that ties social scientists to health activists in new ways. Recognizing the ways in which arbitration over what counts as "science" and what gets relegated to the category of "non-science" is a second contribution, and one that positions health activists to make the case for health over science in some instances. Finally, recognizing the potential erasures that come from a focus on standardizing scientific rigor in producing an evidence-based global health is a third contribution that might be a place for thinking through what it would mean to be "against global health."

In the first era of international health development, it was considered a great achievement to link the notion of health with all development. It was an achievement that constructed a nexus of health and science, as well as connected the sciences of economics, engineering, and demography to health. In the recent turn to global health sciences, the health/science nexus has itself been displaced by an urgent sense of the need for more scientific rigor in all of these endeavors. It is in this last shift that it is possible to see how being "against global health" might be productive in efforts to achieve health.

NOTES

1. Thanks to Jonathan Metzl for including my work in this volume and for his editing suggestions, and to the Institute on Global Conflict and Cooperation for providing the funding through which some of this work was realized. This article was originally presented as a paper at the 107th Annual Meeting of the American Anthropological Association, November 19–23, 2008, in San Francisco, California. The session title was "Collaborations, Experiments and Care: At the Frontier of Science and Medicine."

2. See Theodore M. Brown, Marcos Cueto, and Elizabeth Fee, "The World Health Organization and the Transition from 'International' to 'Global' Public Health," *American Journal of Public Health* 96, no. 1 (January 2006): 62–72.

3. For the final report on this conference, see Vincanne Adams, Thomas E. Novotny, and Hannah Leslie, "Global Health Diplomacy," *Medical Anthropology: Cross-Cultural Studies in Health and Illness* 27, no. 4 (2008): 315–23.

4. See Vinh-Kim Nguyen, "Antiretroviral Globalism: Biopolitics and Therapeutic Citizenship," in *Global Assemblages: Technology, Politics, and Ethics as Anthropological Problems*, ed. Aihwa Ong and Stephen J. Collier (Malden, MA: Blackwell, 2005), 124–44, and Stacy Leigh Pigg, "Languages of Sex and AIDS in Nepal: Notes on the Social Production of Commensurability," *Cultural Anthropology* 16, no. 4 (November 2001): 481–541.

5. See George Foster, "Relationships between Theoretical and Applied Anthropology: A Public Health Program Analysis," *Human Organization* 11, no. 3 (1952): 5–16. See also works by Carl E. Taylor, including "Hindu Medicine and India's Health," *Atlantic Monthly* 190, no. 1 (1952): 38–42.

6. See Warwick Anderson and Vincanne Adams, "Pramoedya's Chickens: Postcolonial Studies of Technoscience," in *The Handbook of Science and Technology Studies, 3rd ed.*, ed. Edward J. Hackett (Cambridge: MIT Press, 2007).

7. See E. Richard Brown, "Public Health and Imperialism: Early Rockefeller Programs at Home and Abroad," in *The Cultural Crisis of Modern Medicine*, ed. John Ehrenreich (New York: Monthly Review Press, 1978), 252–70.

8. See Warwick Anderson, *Colonial Pathologies: American Tropical Medicine, Race, and Hygiene in the Philippines* (Durham: Duke University Press, 2006) and Megan Vaughan, *Curing their Ills: Colonial Power and African Illness* (Cambridge: Polity Press, 1991).

9. See Gyan Prakash, *Another Reason: Science and the Imagination of Modern India* (Princeton: Princeton University Press, 1999).

10. For more examples of such cases, see articles in David Landy, ed., *Culture, Disease, and Healing: Studies in Medical Anthropology* (New York: Macmillan, 1977).

11. See Lola Romanucci-Ross, Daniel E. Moerman, and Laurence R. Tancredi, *The Anthropology of Medicine: From Culture to Method* (New York: Praeger, 1983); Michael H. Logan and Edward E. Hunt, eds., *Health and the Human Condition: Perspectives on Medical Anthropology* (North Scituate, MA: Duxbury Press, 1978); and Robert S. Desowitz, *New Guinea Tapeworms and Jewish Grandmothers: Tales of Parasites and People* (New York: Norton, 1981).

12. See Frantz Fanon, "Medicine and Colonialism," in Ehrenreich, *Cultural Crisis*, 229–51.

13. See, for example, E. E. Evans-Pritchard, *Witchcraft, Oracles and Magic among the Azande* (Oxford: Clarendon Press, 1976).

14. Led by Carl E. Taylor, Johns Hopkins University was a lead institution in this process in the United States.

15. See Benjamin D. Paul, *Health, Culture, and Community: Case Studies of Public Reactions to Health Programs* (New York: Russell Sage Foundation, 1955).

16. See Stacy Leigh Pigg, "Globalizing the Facts of Life," in "Sex and Development: Science, Sexuality, and Morality in Global Perspective," ed. Vincanne Adams and Stacy Leigh Pigg (Durham: Duke University Press, 2005), 39–66.

17. See my "Saving Tibet? An Inquiry into Modernity, Lies, Truths, and Belief," *Medical Anthropology* 24, no. 1 (2005): 71–110.

18. See Mark Nichter and Mimi Nichter, *Anthropology and International Health: Asian Case Studies* (Amsterdam: Gordon and Breach, 1996).

19. Such studies have a long history, from Foster, "Relationships" and Paul, *Health, Culture, and Community* to more contemporary work.

20. See Nancy Scheper-Hughes, *Death Without Weeping: The Violence of Everyday Life in Brazil* (Berkeley: University of California Press, 1992).

21. See Peter J. Brown, "Microparasites and Macroparasites," *Cultural Anthropology* 2, no. 1 (February 1987): 155–71.

22. This was an irony for the workshop on global health diplomacy since political issues such as these become obstacles to policy reform and to the creation of treaties.

23. See Joao Biehl, "Drugs for All: The Future of Global AIDS Treatment," *Medical Anthropology* 27, no. 2 (2008): 99–105, and Adriana Petryna, Andrew Lakoff, and Arthur Kleinman, eds., *Global Pharmaceuticals: Ethics, Markets, Practices* (Durham: Duke University Press, 2006).

24. See Adriana Petryna, *When Experiments Travel: Clinical Trials and the Global Search for Human Subjects* (Princeton: Princeton University Press, 2009).

25. See Ian Whitmarsh, *Biomedical Ambiguity: Race, Asthma, and the Contested Meaning of Genetic Research in the Caribbean* (Ithaca: Cornell University Press, 2008).

26. See Lawrence Cohen, "Where it Hurts: Indian Material for an Ethics of Organ Transplantation," *Deadalus* 128, no. 4 (Fall 1999): 135–65.

27. Conversation with author, April 2009, Xining China.

28. Conversation with author, 2003, Lhasa, Tibetan Autonomous Region, China.

29. Pierre Buekens, Gerald Keusch, Jose Belizan, and Zulfiqar Ahmed Bhutta, "Evidence-Based Global Health," *JAMA* 291, no. 21 (June 2, 2004): 2639–41.

30. Quoted in Jon Cohen, "The New World of Global Health," *Science* 311, no. 5758 (January 13, 2006): 163.

31. See Judith Justice, *Policies, Plans, and People: Culture and Health Development in Nepal* (Berkeley: University of California Press, 1986).

32. Buekens et al., "Evidence-Based Global Health," 2639.

33. Rupert Kaul, Joshua Kimani, Nico J. Nagelkerke et al., "Monthly Antibiotic Chemoprophylaxis and Incidence of Sexually Transmitted Infections and HIV-1 Infection in Kenyan Sex Workers: A Randomized Controlled Trial," *JAMA* 291, no. 21 (June 2, 2004): 2555–62.

34. Elaine L. Larson, Susan X. Lin, Cabilla Gomez-Pichardo, and Phyllis Della-Latta, "Effect of Antibacterial Home Cleaning and Handwashing Products on Infectious Disease Symptoms: a Randomized, Double-Blind Trial," *Annals of Internal Medicine* 140, no. 5 (March 2, 2004): 321–29.

35. Juan A. Rivera, Daniela Sotres-Alvarez, Jean-Piere Habicht, Teresa Shamah, and Salvador Villalpando, "Impact of the Mexican Program for Education, Health, and Nutrition (Progresa) on Rates of Growth and Anemia in Infants and Young Children: A Randomized Effectiveness Study," *JAMA* 291, no. 21 (June 2, 2004): 2563.

36. Buekens et al., "Evidence-Based Global Health," 2639.

37. Ibid., 2640.

38. The Bill and Melinda Gates Foundation, "Gates Foundation Launches $100 Million Initiative to Spur Innovation in Global Health Resarch," Press Release, October 9, 2007; see also Robert Walgate, "Gates Foundation Picks 14 Grand Challenges For Global Disease Research," *Bulletin of the World Health Organization* 81, no. 12 (March 1, 2004): 915–16.

39. There are countercurrents within global health sciences. Groups like the Boston-based Partners in Health stand at the edge of this rising tyranny, keeping the priority on outreach, the delivery of services, the provision of care, and the prioritization of the poor. Using an explicitly human rights approach to health care, the organization spends less effort on designing randomized clinical studies of outcomes than on ensuring the production of a workforce that attends to relentless caregiving beyond the clinic. These efforts, however, are vulnerable to the criticisms of being "loosey-goosey" when it comes to documenting results because they do not generate the same kinds of scientific data as do randomized trials in the world of evidence-based accountability.

40. For example, the new cohort of master's degree students in Global Health Sciences at UCSF have proposed research projects like the following: a randomized controlled trial to determine the effectiveness of an educational intervention in basic neonatal care in improving neonatal health outcomes as compared to regular care; a comparative economic analysis of the cost-effectiveness of using insecticide-treated bednets versus indoor residual spraying for malaria in high endemicity areas; and a randomized controlled trial of the improvements in health and nutrition among HIV-positive farmers in Kenya.

Part II

Seeing Health through Morality

5

The Social Immorality of
Health in the Gene Age

Race, Disability, and Inequality

DOROTHY ROBERTS

The expansion of genetic research and technologies has helped to create a new "biological citizenship" that enables individuals to take unprecedented authority over their health at the molecular level. Preimplantation genetic diagnosis (PGD), for example, allows parents to select embryos that are shown by genetic testing to be free from hundreds of genetic conditions. Genetic scientists are developing "personalized medicine" which will treat diseases by matching drugs to each individual's unique genetic profile. Web-based biotech companies already offer to genotype DNA sent to them by customers and provide personalized reports about their ancestry and risk for various conditions. According to British sociologist Nikolas Rose, "Our very biological life itself has entered the domain of decision and choice."[1] Some celebrate biocitizenship because it enhances human agency as patients "become active and responsible consumers of medical services and products ranging from pharmaceuticals to reproductive technologies and genetic tests" and are empowered to form alliances with physicians, scientists, and clinicians to advocate for their interests.[2]

Debates about the ethics of these biotechnologies that enable biocitizenship often pit health against social justice. Disability rights critics argue, for example, that addressing discrimination against the disabled by selecting out embryos predicted to have undesirable genetic conditions devalues the lives of people currently living with disabilities and further ignores the social barriers they encounter. Biotech advocates deploy the priority of good health to deflect concerns about the power of these technologies to reinforce race, gender, and other social inequities. They portray health as the unassailable aim of human biotechnologies and insist that it takes precedence over political and social interests. According to this view, health trumps social justice.

Ethical debates about genetic selection technologies and race-specific pharmaceuticals illustrate health's social immorality in the gene age. Racial medicine's promoters argue that the health benefits of racially specific drugs outweigh their harmful potential to reify race as a biological category. Similarly, arguments in favor of preimplantation genetic diagnosis place the reducing of genetic risk above concerns about the procedure's impact on the social status of women and people with disabilities. But how should we respect the dignity and rights of those people who carry a genetic trait that would be eradicated by genetic screening and selective abortion or PGD? What about the pressure that many pregnant women feel to undergo genetic testing and to not bear children predicted to have disabilities? How will we keep in view the ways that race, class, and gender inequities contribute to health disparities?

I am against a conception of biocitizenship that uses health as a shield against claims for social justice. This view pretends that health can be divorced from its sociopolitical context, and it ignores the ways in which new biotechnologies shape and are shaped by social power. Moreover, reliance on citizens' personal consumption of biotechnology to address social inequities only supports the neoliberal shift of responsibility for public welfare from the state to the private realms of individual, family, and market. Letting health trump social justice does not really improve the welfare of most people; it supports the interests of big business and the most privileged members of society. It creates a false dichotomy between health and justice that hides the social factors that determine health not only for individuals, but for the entire nation. Debates about the ethics of race-specific drugs and genetic selection technologies illustrate the social immorality of arguments that use health to conceal these technologies' potential to promote inequality. These technologies stem from a medical model that attributes problems caused by social inequities to each individual's genetic makeup and that holds individuals, rather than the public, responsible for fixing these inequities. A more just society would be a healthier one.

Race and Personalized Medicine

Genetic scientists promise to soon develop personalized medicine, which will enable each biocitizen to predict, diagnose, and treat illnesses according to his or her own unique genome.[3] Researchers in the field of pharmacogenomics, which studies the genetic origins of disease and differential responses to medications, are developing "tailored" drugs that are safer and more effective than conventional medicines. Until individualized gene mapping is available, however, race increasingly serves as a proxy for genetic variation.[4] In other words, some researchers use the race of patients to guess what genes they have. The first step toward personalized medicine has been the production of pharmaceuticals designed to treat diseases in particular racial and ethnic groups. Of course, tailoring medical therapies to individual patients is an amazing scientific innovation. If race works to facilitate that tailoring, why not make use of it to treat people who are sick? A careful look at the role of race in developing drugs for specific groups, however, raises serious concerns about its social consequences.

In June 2005, the Food and Drug Administration approved the first race-based pharmaceutical, BiDil, to treat heart failure in African Americans.[5] BiDil is the combination into a single pill of two generic drugs that doctors were already prescribing to patients regardless of race. Yet the FDA permitted its maker, Nitromed, to market BiDil as a race-specific drug based on the results of a clinical trial composed entirely of self-identified African American patients. Making BiDil race-specific allowed Nitromed to extend its patent to the year 2020, giving the company market exclusivity and the potential for huge profits on sales of the drug.[6] The unproven theory underlying the development of race-specific therapy argues that the reason for higher mortality rates among African American heart patients lies in straightforward biological differences that contribute to the incidence of heart disease or that lead to particular responses to heart medications.

In a March 2001 press release, Nitromed explained that BiDil works especially well for African Americans because "observed racial disparities in mortality and therapeutic response rates in black patients may be due in part to ethnic differences in the underlying pathophysiology of heart failure."[7] The FDA also relied on race as a proxy for the underlying genetic mechanism that explains BiDil's effectiveness. In a January 2007 article in *Annals of Internal Medicine*, two FDA doctors presented the agency's perspective: "We hope that further research elucidates the genetic or other factors that predict the usefulness of hydralazine hydrochloride-isosorbide dinitrate [the ingredients in BiDil]. Until then, we are pleased that one defined group has access to a dramatically life-prolonging therapy."[8] Scientists who view race as a surrogate for identifying actual genetic variation in individuals position race-specific drugs as an important step toward personalized medicine. One day, they promise, pharmaceuticals will be tailored according to each patient's individual genotype. But until then, race stands in as a crude approximation.

Prominent African American scientists, doctors, and advocates endorsed BiDil to redress past discrimination against African Americans in medical treatment and access to health care.[9] African Americans had been victims of both medical abuse, such as the infamous syphilis study in Tuskegee, Alabama, and medical neglect. The clinical trial to test the efficacy of BiDil in treating heart failure in African Americans was cosponsored by the Association of Black Cardiologists and supported by the National Medical Association and members of the Black Congressional Caucus. They argued that BiDil fulfilled a long-standing demand that science attend to the particular needs of African Americans who historically had been excluded from good medical care and clinical trials while suffering disproportionately from heart disease. African American support for BiDil illustrates how claims about justice in scientific research have shifted away from protecting socially disadvantaged subjects from unethical practices and toward promoting access to clinical trials and biotech products.[10] At the same time, the pharmaceutical industry now sees African Americans and other people of color as profitable markets in its search for new drugs and as test populations to meet the exploding demand for human subjects and sources of human tissue. It seems scientists have gone from ignoring African American people in medical research and exploiting them as experimental subjects to pitching race-specific drugs to them. While inclusion of diverse groups in biomedical research is important, we must ask if the new focus on racially specific medicine has its own pitfalls.

Genomic studies of human variation like the Human Genome Project have confirmed social scientists' conclusion that race is an invented political category by showing high levels of genetic similarity within the human species.[11] There is more genetic variation within so-called races than between them. Some scholars believe that the science of human genetic diversity will replace race as the preeminent means of grouping people for scientific purposes.[12] By incorporating invented racial groupings into genetic research, scientists and entrepreneurs are producing biotechnologies that validate the belief that race is a natural classification.[13] A renewed trust in inherent racial differences provides a convenient but false explanation for persistent inequities despite the end of de jure discrimination. It is also the perfect complement to social policies that implement the claim that racism has ceased to be the cause of African Americans' unequal status. Race consciousness in social programs like affirmative action is under assault at the very moment that race consciousness in medicine is ascending.

In the face of these concerns, supporters defend race-based pharmaceuticals on grounds that their health benefits outweigh their power to reinforce race as a biological category. At one end of the political spectrum, conservatives who claim that racial differences are real at the genetic level charge their critics with relying on political ideology rather than science.[14] They argue that race is a natural category that became politicized only in the last few decades as a result of post–civil rights identity politics. This ignores the real origins of racial classifications that accommodated European, and later American, imperialism and slavery—the quintessential example of using science to achieve political ends. Conservatives point to racial medicine as scientific confirmation of racial differences that liberals have denied in order to be politically correct.

Sally Satel, a fellow at the American Enterprise Institute, has long defended the use of race in medical practice in response to biological differences between members of different racial groups. In a 2002 *New York Times Magazine* article, "I Am a Racially Profiling Doctor," she concluded, "It is evident that disease is not colorblind, and therefore doctors should not be either."[15] Not surprisingly, Satel supports race-specific pharmaceuticals. "Social race is the phenomenon constructionists have in mind. . . . Biological race, however, is what BiDil's developers are concerned with—that is, race as ancestry."[16] According to this view, racial differences are real at the molecular level, but merely constructed in society; therefore, doctors and researchers cannot be color-blind, but social policy should be. Genomic science, conservatives argue, now gives people license to act on biological differences between races to better understand their health and identities. In this ingenious twist of political logic, those who criticize racial medicine because of its social impact are seen as interfering with health on the basis of racial ideology.

On the other end of the political spectrum, some African American activists also use the concept of health to dismiss social justice objections to race-specific pharmaceuticals. Gary Puckrein, executive director of the National Minority Health Month Foundation, has championed BiDil as an important response to high rates of heart disease among African Americans. Although he acknowledged "[c]oncern about the medical and scientific validity of the concept of race," he dismissed such concern as, "under present circumstances, impractical."[17] In other words, the urgency of addressing the African American health crisis with race-specific drugs overrides objections that race is a social grouping. When I stated at an April 2006 conference at MIT that there was no consensus among African Americans on the benefits of race-based medicine, an NAACP representative in the audience stood up and emotionally disagreed. He argued that support for BiDil by the NAACP and other African American organizations demonstrates a clear consensus in favor of race-specific drugs. He castigated me for jeopardizing African American people's lives by raising criticism of the product.

These African American activists with ties to the pharmaceutical industry stifle criticism of racial medicine by portraying objections as roadblocks to African Americans' access to lifesaving treatment. They position themselves as the exclusive guardians of African American people's health and portray those who express social concerns as the opponents of this health. No critic of race-specific medicine seeks to deny lifesaving drugs to African American people.[18] We simply see no justification for marketing them according to race, and worry about their potential to divert attention away from more significant social reasons for health disparities. Studying and eliminating the social determinants of health inequities is a far more promising course than searching for race-specific genetic difference.

Reprogenetics, Gender, and Disability Rights

In the gene age, biocitizens will manage their health not only by treating genetic illness with personalized medicine, but by eliminating genetic risk altogether. Advanced reproductive technologies that combine assisted conception with genetic selection, or "reprogenetics," allow parents to reduce their children's genetic risk.[19] With preimplantation genetic diagnosis, clinicians take a single-cell biopsy from early embryos, diagnose it for the risk of hundreds of genetic conditions, and select for implantation only those embryos at low risk for these conditions. As Reprogenetics, a New Jersey genetics laboratory that specializes in PGD, puts it, this technique allows for the "replacement to the patient of those embryos classified by genetic diagnosis as normal."[20] Many people see genetic selection technologies as unquestionably good because they improve individuals' chances for good health.[21]

Disability rights activists have pointed out that prenatal and preimplantation genetic diagnosis reinforces the view that "disability itself, not societal discrimination against people with disabilities, is the problem to be solved."[22] This medicalized approach to disability assumes that difficulties experienced by disabled people are caused by physiological limitations that prevent them from functioning normally in society.[23] Although disabilities cause various degrees of impairment, the main hardship experienced by most people with disabilities stems from pervasive discrimination.

Locating the problem inside the disabled body rather than in the social oppression of disabled people leads to eliminating these bodies as the chief solution to impairment. By selecting out disabling traits, these technologies can divert attention away from social arrangements, government policies, and cultural norms that help to define disability and make having disabled children undesirable.[24] Genetic selection is also discriminatory in that it reduces individual children to certain genetic traits that by themselves are deemed sufficient reasons to terminate an otherwise wanted pregnancy or discard an embryo that might otherwise have been implanted.[25]

Reprogenetics also imposes new duties on women who are held responsible for ensuring the genetic fitness of their children. Widespread prenatal testing has already generated greater surveillance of pregnant women and assigned them primary accountability for making the "right" genetic decisions. It is now routine for pregnant women to obtain prenatal diagnoses for certain genetic conditions such as Down syndrome or dwarfism.[26] Furthermore, these women are expected to opt for abortion in order to select against disabling traits identified by genetic testing. Although genetic counseling should be nondirective, many counselors show disapproval when patients decide against selective abortion.[27] Brian Skotko's survey of 985 mothers who received post-natal diagnoses of Down syndrome for their children discovered that many of these mothers were chastised by healthcare professionals for not undergoing prenatal testing.[28] As a result of such pressure, many pregnant women now view genetic testing as an important element of responsible mothering.[29]

Liberal notions of reproductive choice obscure the potential for genetic selection technologies to intensify both discrimination against disabled people and the regulation of women's childbearing decisions. Reprogenetics' sponsors defend the fertility industry's immunity from state regulation in the name of reproductive freedom. In his influential book, *Children of Choice*, legal scholar John Robertson argues that the constitutional right to procreative liberty gives presumptive priority to the decision to use reproduction-assisting technologies.[30] He casts assisted reproduction as inherently progressive as it frees human beings who yearn to create children from their subjugation to the "luck of the natural lottery."[31] Robertson concludes that there is almost never enough harm in genetic selection to justify intrusion into an individual's procreative choices. To use Robertson's triumphant imagery, "In nearly every instance, public policy should keep the gateway to technology open, allowing individuals the freedom to enter as they will."[32] He concedes that decisions to clone or genetically debilitate offspring should be subject to state interference because procreative liberty protects "only actions designed to enable a couple to have normal, healthy offspring whom they intend to rear."[33] Robertson dismisses social justice objections by characterizing them as "symbolic" or "deontological" concerns, as opposed to "actual effects" and "consequentialist" concerns.

Thus, according to this view, freedom to ensure fetal health trumps any harmful social impact caused by reprogenetics.

Indeed, some clients of genetic selection services claim moral superiority over women who have abortions for nonselective reasons. In a July 22, 2004, op-ed in the *New York Times*, Barbara Ehrenreich called on women who aborted fetuses based on prenatal diagnosis to support the general right to abortion.[34] She noted that these women sometimes distinguish themselves from women who have "ordinary" abortions. One woman who aborted a fetus with Down syndrome stated, "I don't look at it as though I had an abortion, even though that is technically what it is. There's a difference. I wanted this baby." On a Website for a support group called "A Heart Breaking Choice," a mother who went to an abortion clinic complains, "I resented the fact that I had to be there with all these girls that did not want their babies."

This moral comparison neglects the history of abortion regulation and the role that abortion rights play in women's social equality. Prior to *Roe v. Wade*, states limited women's reproductive freedom by distinguishing between abortions approved by doctors for "therapeutic" reasons and criminalized elective abortions.[35] All of this makes clear that a defense of biocitizens' reliance on genetic selection technologies to improve children's health can impede the progress of women's and disabled people's rights.

Neoliberalism, Social Justice, and Health

Despite its potential to empower patients, biological citizenship also reflects the shift of responsibility for public welfare from the state to the private realms of individual, family, and market. Marketing genetic testing and pharmacogenomic products directly to consumers is big business for private fertility clinics and biotechnology companies. Consequentially, biomedical research and technology have become major sources of capital accumulation, aided by federal patents on genetic information, FDA approval of pharmaceuticals, and public funding of lucrative private research ventures, such as California's stem cell research initiative.

Both race-specific medicine and genetic selection technologies stem from a medical model that attributes problems caused by social inequities to individuals' genetic makeup and holds individuals, rather than the public, responsible for fixing these inequities. In addition to the deregulation that typically occurs in the service of big business, the new duties imposed on women to ensure the genetic fitness of their children constitute a "re-regulation" that supports capital investment in market-based approaches to health care while state investment in public resources shrinks.[36] And while the racial gap in life expectancy widens,[37] owing largely to the government's failure to address structural inequities, the poor health of African Americans opens new markets for pharmaceutical companies. In this way, human biotechnologies can powerfully reinforce privatization, the hallmark of the neoliberal state that seeks to reduce social welfare programs while advancing private sector interests in the market economy.[38] The claim that these technologies improve people's health is a powerful way to deflect concerns about their unjust social impact and central role in the neoliberal agenda.

Genetic science provides valuable tools for biocitizens to better understand and treat illness. But we should be against a conception of biocitizenship that promotes individual health as a way of ignoring larger social inequities. This view sets up a false dichotomy between health and social justice: it treats health and justice as opposing values, weighs them against each other, and declares health the winner. In fact, social hierarchy is the single most important determinant of health. Numerous studies tracking the health of people along the social ladder show that health gradually worsens as socioeconomic status, including race, declines.[39] The United States is unhealthier than its European counterparts, despite spending far more money on genetic research and medical care, because it has more social inequality. The social immorality of biotechnological advances not only will ensure that their benefits are distributed unequally to the most privileged citizens, but will reinforce inequitable social structures and neoliberal political trends that impede social change. Far from competing against health, attending to social justice is essential to improving it in the gene age.

NOTES

1. Nikolas Rose, *The Politics of Life Itself: Biomedicine, Power, and Subjectivity in the Twenty-First Century* (Princeton: Princeton University Press, 2007), 40.

2. Ibid., 4. See also Sarah Franklin and Celia Roberts, *Born and Made: An Ethnography of Preimplantation Genetic Diagnosis* (Princeton: Princeton University Press, 2006).

3. See M. Gregg Bloche, "Race-Based Therapeutics," *New England Journal of Medicine* 351, no. 20 (November 11, 2004): 2035–37.

4. See Sandra Soo-Jin Lee, "Racialized Drug Design: Implications of Pharmacogenomics for Health Disparities," *American Journal of Public Health* 95, no. 12 (2005): 2133–38.

5. See Jonathan Kahn, "Race in a Bottle," *Scientific American* 297, no. 2 (August 2007): 40–45.

6. See Jonathan Kahn, "How a Drug Becomes 'Ethnic': Law, Commerce, and the Production of Racial Categories in Medicine," *Yale Journal of Health Policy, Law and Ethics* 4 (2004): 1–46.

7. NitroMed, "NitroMed Receives FDA Letter on BiDil NDA, a Treatment for Heart Failure in Black Patients," Press Release, March 8, 2001, http://www.nitromed.com/press/03-08-01.html; NitroMed, "NitroMed Initiates Confirmatory BiDil Trial in African American Heart Failure Patients," Press Release, March 17, 2001, http://www.nitromed.com/press/03-17-01.html.

8. Robert Temple and Norman L. Stockbridge, "BiDil for Heart Failure in Black Patients: The US Food and Drug Administration Perspective," *Annals of Internal Medicine* 146, no. 1 January-February 2007): 61.

9. Dorothy E. Roberts, "Is Race-Based Medicine Good for Us?: African-American Approaches to Race, Biotechnology, and Equality," Journal of Law, Medicine and Ethics 36 (2008): 537–45.

10. See Steven Epstein, *Inclusion: The Politics of Difference in Medical Research* (Chicago: University of Chicago Press, 2007).

11. See Joseph L. Graves, *The Emperor's New Clothes: Biological Theories of Race at the Millennium* (New Brunswick, NJ: Rutgers University Press, 2001).

12. See Jenny Reardon, *Race to the Finish: Identity and Governance in an Age of Genomics* (Princeton: Princeton University Press, 2005); see also Richard Lewontin, *Human Diversity* (Boston: W. H. Freeman, 1995).

13. Troy Duster, "Race and Reification in Science," *Science* 307 (2005): 1050–51.

14. See, for example, Sally Satel, PC, M.D.: *How Political Correctness Is Corrupting Medicine* (New York: Basic Books, 2001); Sally Satel and Jonathan Klick, *The Health Disparities Myth: Diagnosing the Treatment Gap* (Washington, DC: AEI, 2006); and Jon Entine, *Abraham's Children: Race, Identity, and the DNA of the Chosen People* (New York: Grand Central, 2007).

15. Satel, "I Am a Racially Profiling Doctor," *New York Times Magazine*, May 5, 2002, 56.

16. Satel, "Race and Medicine Can Mix Without Prejudice: How the Story of BiDil Illuminates the Future of Medicine," *Medical Progress Today*, December 10, 2004, http://www.medicalprogresstoday.com/spotlight/spotlight_indarchive.php?id=449.

17. Gary Puckrein, "BiDil: From Another Vantage Point," *Health Affairs* 25, no. 5 (2006): w372.

18. See Jonathan Kahn and Pamela Sankar, "Being Specific About Race-Specific Medicine," *Health Affairs* 25, no. 5 (2006): w375–w377.

19. See Erik Parens and Lori P. Knowles, "Reprogenetics and Public Policy: Reflections and Recommendations," in *Reprogenetics: Law, Policy, and Ethical Issues*, ed. Lori P. Knowles and Gregory E. Kaebnick (Baltimore: Johns Hopkins University Press, 2007), 253–94.

20. Reprogenetics, "Everything Associated with Preimplantation Genetic Diagnosis—PGD," http://www.reprogenetics.com/.

21. See Lee M. Silver, *Remaking Eden: How Genetic Engineering and Cloning Will Transform the American Family* (New York: Harper Perennial, 1998); see also Gregory Stock, *Redesigning Humans: Our Inevitable Genetic Future* (New York: Houghton Mifflin, 2002).

22. Erik Parens and Adrienne Asch, "The Disability Rights Critique of Prenatal Genetic Testing: Reflections and Recommendations," in *Prenatal Testing and Disability Rights*, ed. Erik Parens and Adrienne Asch (Washington, DC: Georgetown University Press, 2007), 13.

23. Marsha Saxton, "Why Members of the Disability Community Oppose Prenatal Diagnosis and Selective Abortion," in Parens and Asch, *Prenatal Testing*, 149.

24. Susan Wendell, *The Rejected Body: Feminist Philosophical Reflections on Disability* (New York: Routledge, 1996), 35–56.

25. See Adrienne Asch, "Why I Haven't Changed my Mind about Prenatal Diagnosis: Reflections and Refinements," in Parens and Asch, *Prenatal Testing*, 234–58.

26. See Cynthia M. Powell, "The Current State of Prenatal Genetic Testing in the United States," in Parens and Asch, *Prenatal Testing*, 44–53.

27. See David T. Helm, Sara Miranda, and Naomi Angoff Chedd, "Prenatal Diagnosis of Down Syndrome: Mothers' Reflections on Supports Needed from Diagnosis to Birth," *Mental Retardation* 36, no. 1 (February 1998): 55–61.

28. See Brian Skotko, "Mothers of Children with Down Syndrome Reflect on Their Postnatal Support," *Pediatrics* 115, no. 1 (January 2005): 64–77.

29. Amy Harmon, "THE WORLD; Genetic Testing + Abortion = ???," *New York Times*, May 13, 2007, Week in Review Section, Midwest Edition.

30. John A. Robertson, *Children of Choice: Freedom and the New Reproductive Technologies* (Princeton: Princeton University Press, 1994). See also John A. Robertson, "Extending Preimplantation Genetic Diagnosis: The Ethical Debate," *Human Reproduction* 18, no. 3 (March 2003): 465–71. For an extended critique of *Children of Choice*, see Dorothy E. Roberts, "Social Justice, Procreative Liberty, and the Limits of Liberal Theory: Robertson's Children of Choice," *Law & Social Inquiry* 20, no. 4 (Autumn 1995): 1005–21.

31. Robertson, *Children of Choice*, 2.

32. Ibid., 221.

33. Ibid., 167.

34. Barbara Ehrenreich, "Owning Up to Abortion," *New York Times*, July 22, 2004, Opinion Section, Midwest Edition.

35. See Johanna Schoen, *Choice and Coercion: Birth Control, Sterilization, and Abortion in Public Health and Welfare* (Chapel Hill: University of North Carolina Press, 2005), 153–86.

36. See Roxanne Mykitiuk, "The New Genetics in the Post-Keynesian State," Canadian Women's Health Network, http://www.cwhn.ca/groups/biotech/availdocs/15-mykitiuk.pdf.

37. Robert Pear, "Gap in Life Expectancy Widens for the Nation," *New York Times*, March 23, 2008, U.S. Section, Midwest Edition.

38. See David Harvey, *A Brief History of Neoliberalism* (New York: Oxford University Press, 2007).

39. See Donald A. Barr, *Health Disparities in the United States: Social Class, Race, Ethnicity, and Health* (Baltimore: Johns Hopkins University Press, 2008); See also Evelyn M. Kitagawa and Philip M. Hauser, *Differential Mortality in the United States: A Study in Socioeconomic Epidemiology* (Cambridge, MA: Harvard University Press, 1973); Nancy E. Adler and David H. Rehkopf, "U.S. Disparities in Health: Descriptions, Causes, and Mechanisms," *Annual Review of Public Health* 29 (April 2008): 235–52; Jean-Michel Etienne, Ali Skalli, and Ioannis Theodossiou, "Do Economic Inequalities Harm Health?: Evidence from Europe," Centre for European Labour Market Research, http://auraserv.abdn.ac.uk:9080/aura/bitstream/2164/131/1/ISSN+0143-07-13.pdf; M. G. Marmot, M. Kogevinas, and M. A. Elston, "Social/Economic Status and Disease," *Annual Review of Public Health* 8 (May 1987): 111–35.

6

Fat Panic and the New Morality

KATHLEEN LEBESCO

Medicine is a major institution of social control. The United States is religious, but out-and-out rebukes of "heathen!" or "sinner!" to disorderly behavior don't exactly fly at the present moment. Instead, the language of health and risk has become a repository for a new kind of moralism. There's been much talk lately about the extent to which morals are in sharp decline as evidenced by phenomena as disparate as public rudeness, high crime rates, dips in attendance at organized religious services, and our increasing reliance on scientific perspectives in matters of the body. As a researcher of the politics of fatness in U.S. culture for the last ten years, I beg to differ with those who say morals are on the wane. In fact, obsessions over sliding morals in a neoliberal context have turned many of us into moral scolds. When arbiters of this morality like *Men's Fitness* name Houston, Las Vegas, Detroit, or Honolulu some of the "fattest cities in America," local public health officials recruit the participation of urban inhabitants in "Shape Up, America!" campaigns, trying desperately to unseat themselves of this dire designation by using tactics of guilt and fear.[1] New York, Washington, Arkansas, Vermont, and Nebraska have all recently seen "Twinkie taxes" debated in their state legislatures;[2] they are most often defeated by business-friendly politicians who argue that the moral responsibility for restraint should be with the consumer and that taxes ultimately punish industry.[3] Fat people are chided for their weight by mere acquaintances and passers-by on a daily basis; they are exhorted to eat less and better, and to move more. Newspaper editorials and reality television shows condemn fat airline passengers whose imagined sloth and gluttony crowds their seat-row neighbors.[4] Instead of jumping on the "declining morals" bandwagon, what I want to think about is how the deployment of moral injunctions is in full force when it comes to fatness. I will outline what a "moral panic" is, explain how the "obesity epidemic" fits well within this paradigm, and evaluate the responses to this supposed epidemic that have been generated in public discourse.

Sociologist Stanley Cohen, popularizer of the concept of a "moral panic" first articulated by Marshall McLuhan, argues that the objects of panics are both new and old; they are both damaging in themselves and merely warning signs of something more ominous; they are transparent yet opaque. In a nutshell, Cohen argues that moral panics are "condensed political struggles to control the means of cultural reproduction."[5] Moral panics are marked by *concern* about an imagined threat; *hostility* in the form of moral outrage toward individuals and agencies responsible for the problem; *consensus* that something must be done about the serious threat; *disproportionality* in reports of harm; and *volatility* in terms of the eruption of panic. Finally, according to Cohen, "successful moral panics owe their appeal to their ability to find points of resonance with wider anxieties."[6]

Panic about fatness finds itself expressed in contemporary rhetoric about the "obesity epidemic." There is no shortage of *concern* about the imagined threat of fatness: headlines trumpet its alleged consequences every day. In a recent week, I saw the following headlines plastered across newspapers: "Obesity Could be the Biggest Threat to Female Fertility" (London *Daily Mail*), "Obese at the Age of Two; Fears of a 'Fat Time Bomb' as an Increasing Number of Children Need Medical Help with Weight Issues" (London *Daily Mail*), and "Fat Chance for the Overweight: Insurance: Beware—the Cost of Life and Critical Health Cover is Set to Expand in Line with Your Waist Measurement" (*The Guardian*). TV shows like *The Biggest Loser* and *Celebrity Fit Club* personalize the concern. In the medical world, we are warned of soaring rates of diabetes and heart disease, not to mention plain old death. In the economic realm, we are cautioned about the financial costs of fatness from insurance rates, lost work days, and slumping worker productivity. In the media, we are invited to scoff at celebrities who dare to gain a few pounds, just as we are reminded that they have fallen out of favor with our seemingly timeless notions of beauty and sexiness.

We also direct a great deal of *hostility* in the form of moral outrage at the presumed agents of the "obesity epidemic." For the most part, that means we point the finger at individuals who we understand to be lazy, out of control, without will, ignorant, or some combination thereof. A small minority of critics choose instead to place the blame for our expanding waistlines on larger social structures, citing government subsidies of unhealthful food products, a profit-hungry fast food industry, car culture, suburbanization, and minimal physical demands in the information and service economy. At other times, bad parenting (usually read as bad mothering) is blamed for making our children fatter. Women who work outside of the home (and thus are less available to cook nutritious, balanced meals) and those who use the television as a babysitter, thus encouraging a sedentary lifestyle in their offspring, are framed as the scourges of civilization. Whether the individual or the larger structure is targeted, the tone is typically hostile and morally righteous: "How *dare* they!"

Consensus that something must be done about the "obesity epidemic" is easy to come by; even the individual-blamers and the society-blamers are united in their conviction that something has got to give. What actually *should* be done is another matter. Will we have more success in reducing obesity rates if we shame people about their weight and exhort them to modify their diets and increase their rates of exercise? Or do we begin to fix the problem by putting in sidewalks, making healthy food affordable, and haranguing fast food outlets into changing their business practices and menus? Either way something has got to give, say the proponents of "obesity epidemic" rhetoric. It's the rare bird outside of fat activists and researchers (who instead highlight the inhabitability of fat bodies even in light of exaggerated morbidity and mortality statistics for fat people) who departs from this logic.

Furthermore, reports of the harm caused by fatness are *disproportional*. Readers of most interpretations of medical data in the popular press would find the existence of a healthy fat person remarkable, I think. To riff on Mark Twain, rumors of our deaths have been greatly exaggerated. In a 2006 article in the *International Journal of Epidemiology*, Paul Campos and his colleagues convincingly undermine empirical claims made on behalf of the "obesity epidemic," including those that see obesity as a major cause of mortality, that see fatness as pathological, and that see weight loss as good and practical.[7] For instance, Campos and colleagues find that "among the obese, little or no increase in relative risk for premature mortality is observed until one reaches BMIs in the upper 30s or higher. In other words, the vast majority of people labeled 'overweight' and 'obese' according to current definitions do not in fact face any meaningful increased risk for early death."[8] They also problematize statistical linkages between body mass and mortality because of failures to consider confounding factors like fitness, exercise, diet quality, and family history. Their findings suggest a distinct lack of proportion between the hype surrounding obesity and the lived experience of fatness.

The concern over the "obesity epidemic" has also been highly *volatile*. In a recent study, Abigail Saguy and Kevin Riley trace the moment that the fat fire ignited. Around 1994, news outlets looking for enticing stories—stories that appear to affect all of us—began printing stories interpreting medical research about obesity for a wider audience. The number of those stories multiplied exponentially. A Lexis-Nexis search for the phrase "obesity epidemic" in the general news of major newspapers in English-speaking countries in 1993 shows exactly one hit; that number grows so explosively that by 2001, there are 101 hits and by 2004, 770 hits. This is but a tiny fragment of all news pieces in the public arena in these years, but it effectively represents the explosion of interest in the "obesity epidemic."

Fat panic appears to be partly borne out of moral injunctions against sloth and gluttony in Judeo-Christian culture. Fat-hating author Michael Fumento criticizes fat activists, suggesting that they have "turned what had been two of the Seven Deadly Sins—sloth and gluttony—into a right and a badge of honor."[9] I might point out that our culture has less of an issue with slothful people who happen to be thin (and there are plenty) and gluttons who don't wear the visual evidence of their appetites on their bodies (because of high metabolisms or bulimia or a host of other reasons). Of course, the biblical injunctions are against the actions rather than the actors in this "love the sinner, hate the sin" mentality, but translated into a moral code for everyday life, the body of the actor becomes the site of the problem. Thin or average-sized people are not disciplined for sloth or gluttony the same way that fat people are. Moreover, fat people can sometimes buy themselves some breathing room from accusations of moral turpitude by distracting attention away from their bodies toward their good faith efforts to be something other than fat.

Fat panic took flight in the late '90s precisely because it resonates with wider anxieties in our present culture about race, class, and sex. Gone are the days of scarce and unpredictable resources when fatness signified wealth, status, and leisure. Fatness in our present time of abundance in the United States is now more closely associated with the poor and working classes. If African Americans and Latinos are fatter than whites and Asians, and women are more likely than men to be fat, fatness haunts us as a reminder of deteriorating physical privilege in terms of race and sex.[10] It does not surprise me that fatness begins to be framed as an epidemic based on social biases against those we imagine to be indolent and undisciplined only after it becomes more associated with women, the poor, and people of color than wealthy white men. In his writing on governmentality, Mitchell Dean sees a fluid division between active citizens who can manage their own risk and targeted populations who require intervention. Risks associated with obesity seem aimed at "reinscribing and recoding earlier languages of stratification, disadvantage, and marginalization."[11] This historical trajectory upholds the contention of

Australian researchers Michael Gard and Jan Wright that obsession over the consequences of fatness is misguided in that the "dire predictions" associated with fatness have "more to do with preconceived moral and ideological beliefs about fatness than a sober assessment of existing evidence."[12]

I have spent several years as a researcher tracking critical responses to the deployment of "obesity epidemic" research in public discourse and assessing the political usefulness of the strategies employed by those who won't simply buy in to the hype. The hearts of these critics are often in the right place—they want to make the world safe for fat people who suffer discrimination, ridicule, and harassment—but often their strategies are problematic and beg closer consideration. Arguments that seek to salvage fat people's selfhood are often predicated on ideologically fraught assumptions about the valor of science, the usefulness of pathology, or the inevitable determinism of social structures on individual behavior.

In the present moment, medical arguments about obesity trump political arguments about the relationship of fatness to identity, subjectivity, and human rights. Trying to talk about fatness to most "medical-type science persons" (as Jerry Lewis would say) is like banging one's head against a thick, thick wall: even those who acknowledge the political consequences of their demonization of fatness—oppression for fat people and a precarious perch for the rest of us who teeter on the brink of weight gain—play the righteous crusader card and invoke comparisons to illness. Those scholars and activists who attempt to destabilize medical arguments about obesity on scientific rather than political grounds often come off as not terribly credible, given that they are engaged in secondary research, critiquing and reframing both medical research and media reports about this research. There are very few researchers doing primary scientific research on fatness who do not begin from the premise that obesity is a problem, despite their veils of neutral indifference. The master's tools of medical fact are unable to dismantle the house of fat oppression built on a foundation of scientific rhetoric.

Laypeople who want to undo fat oppression often take advantage of medicalized arguments, figuring that pathologizing fatness—proving that one cannot control it—takes the blame off of fat folks. This is a strategy borrowed from gay and lesbian activism, which often promotes the "born that way" explanation for sexual identification as a platform for civil rights. It's often successful in the short run, but I find it particularly dangerous as a political strategy. Medicalizing or pathologizing a condition can help to remove blame from the individual, but I believe that it actually *extends* the reach of moralizing discourse. The strategy is also reminiscent of Stockholm syndrome: what tempts people to make use, as part of emancipatory political projects, of the very same medical discourse that has been used to justify their oppression? Over ten years ago, Wendy Chapkis decried this return to biological determinism as a guarantor of civil rights protection, reminding us that "difference may be arguably described as a 'fact of nature,' but its expression remains a social and political act. That right to enact difference—without relinquishing human and civil rights—can only be collectively won or lost, not partially extended on a case by case basis to those considered deserving by 'the rest of us.'"[13] The fat person who argues moral validity by saying that he can't help being fat and has good eating habits and takes plenty of regular exercise seeks deliverance. It is an understandable goal, but one based on truly fraught reasoning that allows healthism to flourish unchecked. As sociologists Abigail Saguy and Kevin Riley point out, "although a focus on behavior rather than body size potentially removes the stigma associated with larger bodies, it may reinforce the moral imperative to engage in healthy lifestyles."[14]

As I indicated earlier, other contingents focus less on the medical inevitability of fatness and point their fingers instead at larger social structures. Instead of obsessing over personal choice, others like Greg Critser, Morgan Spurlock, and Eric Schlosser want to hold on to the vilification of obesity but shift the blame from the individual to the society.[15] Critser condemns government crop subsidies, while Spurlock and Schlosser denounce the fast food industry. These are illuminating projects, but not particularly politically useful in this context, as they allow human subjectivity to hang in the balance, with the redemption of fat people dependent upon victimization narratives that remove most hints of agency. But then again, remedying fat oppression is not the political game of these authors.

Many within the size acceptance movement advance other structural arguments, such as links between fatness and low socioeconomic status that result in an inability to afford healthy food which further exacerbates fatness. Also popular is a critical assessment of our educational apparatus which instructs people about proper nutrition and offers a patronizing portraiture of fat people (especially those belonging to racial and ethnic minorities) as potentially salvageable should they become enlightened and lose weight. Finally, a focus on the lack of time and space for exercise and movement in our communities and our work-centered lives also buys a bit of breathing room for fat individuals oppressed by the dominant discourse. But swapping out the biological determinist strategies I outlined moments ago for an *environmental* determinist argument is not the best solution, either. It may make the individual less morally suspect, but it does nothing to dismantle the overarching and oppressive moral framework of health.

If imagining the body as a project meshes with core American values, questioning that schema is downright unpatriotic, which explains our former Surgeon General Richard Carmona's equation of obesity with the September 11 terror attacks.[16] Contemporary neoliberal ideologies incite good citizens to take care of their own health; they punish those who fail to live up to this socially constructed moral obligation. I strongly question the political motivations of those who frame our collective slight weight gain as an epidemic, and I bridle at healthist arguments, whether they are used to condemn or to rescue fat people from moral censure.[17] I feel unwilling, however, to throw the baby out with the bath water. To glibly dismiss the material reality of "good health" requires a privileged position. Anybody who has suffered through a debilitating illness knows as much. But what I would like us to do is think about how our insistence on turning efforts to achieve good health into a greater moral enterprise means that health also becomes a sharp political stick with which much harm is ultimately done.

It is tempting to stop short at a theoretical critique of healthism, smug in the knowledge of how moral injunctions invisibly shape concerns about and concepts of health. An alternative to this form of complacency comes in the form of Health at Every Size (HAES), an on-the-ground movement born out of frustration with traditional biomedical perspectives on health that pathologize fatness. HAES proponents, including members of the Association for Size Diversity & Health, promote respect for bodily diversity; value eating practices that balance nutritional needs with hunger, satiety, appetite, and pleasure; and endorse pleasurable, individually appropriate physical activity rather than exercise aimed merely at weight loss.[18] HAES seeks to broaden the definition of health to include typically neglected aspects, including the physical, social, spiritual, occupational, emotional, and intellectual. HAES does not throw health out the window, however. It does not traffic in nihilism, preferring instead a strategy that unmoors the signifier "health" from the morally selective underpinnings on which it now rests. The result is a movement that aims to create well-being without trotting out the old canards that reinforce body prejudices and encourage eating disorders and yo-yo dieting.

As a longtime theorist of fat politics, I engaged with the practical HAES movement for the first time a few years ago on a frustrating workday. Sitting in my office during advisement week, feeling stressed and harried, an email popped up on my computer monitor from the human resources department of my employer, an urban liberal arts college. "Weight Watchers @ Work!" it screamed in bold, colorful letters, addressed to all faculty and staff. A twelve-week program

> designed to accommodate employees' demanding work schedules, At Work takes no more than 45 minutes: the first 15 minutes is for weigh in, followed by a 30 minute topic discussion. Weekly topics will cover behavior modifications, and healthy eating choices. The program will give tips on alleviating stress eating, and creative ways to exercise every day. The goal: tangible results on the road to becoming healthier. All we need is a minimum of 15 employees to pay $168.00. . . .

I felt the blood rush to my face that animals under attack must experience, and the fight-or-flight impulse kicked in. Here was my employer, a bastion of liberal education, not only shilling for the diet industry but extending the very logic—that fatness and health are mutually exclusive—that I had worked so long to unsettle. I had to talk back, but I knew that responding with a sophisticated theoretical critique would miss my mark. People want to be healthy, and who can blame them? What I had here was an opportunity to chop away at the links between fatness and ill health that exist in so many minds. I jumped at it with HAES as my axe.

Mirthful and nervous at the same time, I fired back a reply to all faculty and staff, titling it "Alternative to Weight Watchers at Work":

> Tired of diet pitches on TV? In magazines? In your spam filter and now your inbox? If anyone would prefer to pursue an endeavor that *doesn't* fail 95% of the time, I would be delighted to facilitate a "Health at Every Size" group at MMC. It costs nothing. Weekly topics would cover healthy living in the context of social stigma, pursuing an agenda of true body diversity, understanding that thinness and health are not the same thing, and resisting specious arguments about the efficacy of dieting. Let me know if you're interested!

Then I waited. Over the next few days, dozens of positive responses poured in—people wanted to hear more about this. The Weight Watchers group never materialized due to lack of interest. At our first HAES meeting, nearly twenty employees showed. Some admitted a desire for weight loss that coupled with their curiosity about this new approach. I was prepared for this; Rome wasn't invented in a day, as they say. Others professed such frustration with a lifetime of dieting that they wanted to start toward healthful living with a clean slate and a new attitude. We met weekly, and some members fell away, presumably because they wanted to reach for the standard brass ring of health eschewed by our group. The rest kept coming and started to talk about how cutting down on caffeine helped them to feel well rested, which made them happier to dance or walk or hike during the day. Others related how trying a strategy of eating all their fruits and veggies first in the day made them feel good, almost as good as indulging in some pleasurable sweets later in the day. We went out for walks together in Central Park and plotted world domination.

Lest I paint too rosy a picture, I should mention that certain facets of this HAES experience gave me pause. I was uneasy in the role of expert; I had also hoped that the group would take the general precepts of HAES and run with them, but a structure evolved where I was expected to provide information and make pronouncements on which attitudes toward food, exercise, and the body were truly health-enabling and which were misguided, fat-phobic, or otherwise fraught. As a result, I felt more than a little like the evil twin of the weight-loss group leaders, although I was advancing a rather different agenda. Nikolas Rose writes that "the government of the soul depends upon our recognition of ourselves as ideally and potentially certain sorts of person, the unease generated by a normative judgment of what we are and could become, and the incitement offered to overcome this discrepancy by following the advice of experts in the management of the self."[19] Rose, then, would have me supervising a different stripe of the government of the soul—work that made me antsy. Finally, Alan Petersen and Deborah Lupton point out that "attempts at emancipation, well meaning as they are, often serve to further constrain and disadvantage those individuals to whom they are directed by prescribing specified ways of behaving."[20] For these reasons, I am not absolutely certain that HAES steers clear of *all* the pitfalls of healthism that make me wary. It may be what Toby Miller describes as "unruly subjects seeking to reform themselves," but it avoids enough of them to be a useful tactic in the war on moral terror surrounding health.[21] Even though HAES runs the risk of being implicated in healthism, its goal of disordering traditional notions of health might be a step toward freedom. Where HAES researchers veer into scientific research, I fear that they are buying into conventional modes of resistance; I prefer a playful approach that destabilizes traditional understandings of health. HAES may keep the healthy/sick distinction intact, which is unfortunate, but at least it unhinges sick from fat.

My experience with HAES goes some distance in explaining how people actually respond to discourses of governmentality in their own lives. It certainly showed me how people are capable of reframing the risks that they are trying to avoid. Instead of advancing the notion that fatness means a lack of self-control or signifies a failure of the self to regulate itself, even neophyte HAES folks agree that health should not be a moral enterprise as they come to reject a particular formulation of self-discipline (dieting with the aim of weight loss) that seems essential to citizenship. HAES allows participants to recognize that the public health discourse surrounding obesity is disciplinary, and that its exhortations to individuals to self-monitor and regulate are not always benevolent. It throws a funhouse mirror on the supposedly "healthy body"—the lean, toned body—as a signifier of moral worth. That, it seems to me, is a necessary step toward true health.

NOTES

1. See Eric Huebler, "The Fittest and Fattest Cities in America," *Men's Fitness*, 2008, http://www.mensfitness.com/city_rankings/463, and "Shape Up America! Healthy Weight For Life," *Shape Up America!* http://www.shapeup.org.

2. See Suzanne Leigh, "'Twinkie Tax' Worth a Try in Fight Against Obesity," *USAToday.com*, December 1, 2004, http://www.usatoday.com/news/opinion/editorials/2004-12-01-obesity-edit_x.htm.

3. See "WHO Wants a Fat Tax?" The Center for Consumer Freedom, January 28, 2004, http://www.consumerfreedom.com/news_detail.cfm/headline/2336.

4. See "Airline 'Fat Tax' Call," *The Daily Telegraph*, November 11, 2007, http://www.news.com.au/dailytelegraph/story/0,22049,22736126-5013605,00.html. See also television program *Airline*, producer Nancy Dubuc, A&E Network, 2004–5.

5. Stanley Cohen, *Folk Devils and Moral Panics* (New York: Routledge, 2002), xxxv.

6. Ibid., xxx.

7. Paul Campos, Abigail Saguy, Paul Ernsberger, Eric Oliver, and Glenn Gaesser, "The Epidemiology of Overweight and Obesity: Public Health Crisis or Moral Panic?" *International Journal of Epidemiology* 35, no. 1 (2006): 55.

8. Ibid., 56.

9. Michael Fumento, *The Fat of the Land: Our Health Problem Crisis and How Overweight Americans Can Help Themselves* (New York: Penguin, 1997), 130, cited in Abigail C. Saguy and Kevin W. Riley, "Weighing Both Sides: Morality, Mortality, and Framing Contests over Obesity," *Journal of Health Politics, Policy and Law* 30, no. 5 (October 2005): 885.

10. See "AOA Fact Sheets: Obesity in Minority Populations," American Obesity Association, http://obesity1.tempdomainname.com/subs/fastfacts/Obesity_Minority_Pop.shtml.

11. Mitchell Dean, *Governmentality: Power and Rule in Modern Society* (Thousand Oaks, CA: Sage, 1999), 167.

12. Michael Gard and Jan Wright, *The Obesity Epidemic: Science, Morality, and Ideology* (New York: Routledge, 2005), 3.

13. Wendy Chapkis, "Freaks, Fairies, and Fat Ladies: A Right to Discriminate?" *Critical Sociology* 20, no. 3 (1994): 153.

14. Saguy and Riley, "Weighing Both Sides," 896.

15. See Greg Critser, *Fat Land: How Americans Became the Fattest People in the World* (Boston: Houghton Mifflin, 2003); *Super Size Me*, dir. Morgan Spurlock, DVD, 100 min., Sony Pictures, 2004; and Eric Schlosser, *Fast Food Nation: The Dark Side of the All-American Meal* (Boston: Houghton Mifflin, 2001).

16. See Bob Edwards, "Interview with Surgeon General Richard Carmona," National Public Radio, http: http://www.npr.org/templates/story/story.php?storyId=1524183.

17. See K. M. Flegal, M. D. Carroll, R. J. Kuczmarski, and C. L. Johnson, "Overweight and Obesity in the United States: Prevalence and Trends, 1960–1994," *International Journal of Obesity* 22, no. 1 (January 1998): 39–47.

18. See ASDAH: Association for Size and Diversity Health, http://www.sizediversityandhealth.org/.

19. Nikolas Rose, *Governing the Soul: The Shaping of the Private Self* (New York: Routledge, 1990), 11.

20. Alan Petersen and Deborah Lupton, *The New Public Health: Health and Self in the Age of Risk* (Thousand Oaks, CA: Sage, 1996), 180–81.

21. Toby Miller, *The Well-Tempered Self: Citizenship, Culture, and the Postmodern Subject* (Baltimore: Johns Hopkins University Press, 1993), ix.

7

Against Breastfeeding (Sometimes)

JOAN B. WOLF

I am not against health. I'm also not opposed to freedom. Or compassion. But when one person's freedom to drive her car at any speed infringes on my freedom to travel safely, or when compassion for others leads to a loss of self, I begin to see the merits of restriction and selfishness. I'm troubled by seemingly unobjectionable ideals, including health, when people define them without consideration of the context in which they are pursued, or when they are cultivated with a single-minded zeal that borders on monomania, as in the recent National Breastfeeding Awareness Campaign (NBAC). "You'd never take risks before your baby is born. Why start after?" asked televised public service announcements for the campaign. In one, a pregnant woman is thrown violently from a mechanical bull. In another, two pregnant women square off in a logrolling competition. The message, crafted by the United States Department of Health and Human Services (HHS) and the Ad Council, was clear: formula is dangerous. Only a woman callous enough to compete in extreme sports when pregnant would feed it to her baby, and bottle-feeders are like pregnant women who ride bulls (and presumably get drunk) in bars: they recklessly put their babies at risk. This kind of hyperbole and the campaign's overall message of risk were the result of focus group research indicating that many women believe that breastfeeding provides extra benefits, similar to vitamins, but that formula is standard. NBAC planners saw little point in running a campaign that told women what they already knew. The rhetoric also reflected a widespread American obsession with risk, particularly health risks, and especially health risks to babies and children. Nowadays, people seem to think that risks can be eradicated without cost and that mothers can and should eliminate all imaginable risks to their children. The NBAC made the most of these fantasies. It dramatically misrepresented the research on infant feeding, which does not prove that "breast is best." It distorted the risks associated with formula-feeding and ignored the costs of breastfeeding. And it exploited mothers trying to make good decisions for themselves and their babies. It was, in short, an unethical government attempt to scare women into breastfeeding. I am not against health, but I am opposed to seemingly well-meaning advocates, including the government, presenting health as much simpler than it actually is.

Weak Research

Despite widespread belief to the contrary, science has not demonstrated that breastfeeding is better than formula-feeding for babies. The most respected medical journals are replete with contradictory conclusions about breastfeeding's impact: for every study linking it to better health, another finds it to be irrelevant, weakly significant, or inextricably tied to other unmeasured or unmeasurable factors. With the exception of gastrointestinal (GI) problems, to which I will return at the end of this chapter, the evidence on the health impact of breastfeeding is widely variable for virtually every outcome analyzed, including ear and respiratory infections, cardiovascular disease, obesity, diabetes, cognitive development, leukemia, cancer, pre-term infant health, asthma, allergies, bed-wetting, eczema, growth pains, inflammatory bowel disease, sleep-related breathing disorders, social mobility, stereoacuity, stress, urinary tract infection, and mother-infant bonding. Some research indicates that breastfeeding might actually increase the risk of allergy and asthma for particular children. To be sure, many studies find breastfed babies to be healthier. But many others, some published in the most distinguished journals, find that breastfeeding has no medical benefit. This research is often ignored, downplayed, or misconstrued by scientists stuck in old and increasingly less useful research paradigms, doctors and scientists who lack the time and/or expertise to evaluate the constant barrage of new research, journalists with little to no training in the sciences, and a public largely ignorant of how to interpret scientific evidence.

The research, in a word, is fuzzy. Because breastfeeding is assumed to be medically superior to formula-feeding, scientists consider it unethical to construct randomized controlled trials (RCT) in which babies are randomly assigned to either breast or bottle. Instead, they systematically observe people who have chosen, for their own reasons, to breast or bottle-feed. The results of this "observational" research are often inconsistent with one another, and the ability to replicate such studies is much lower than that for RCTs. One main reason for this is that crucial confounding variables are often not considered in observational studies. Confounding variables are unexamined factors in a study that could plausibly explain the outcome. Potential confounding makes it difficult to isolate the protective powers of breast milk or to rule out the possibility that something associated with breastfeeding is responsible for the benefits attributed to milk itself. For example, if research were to find that most mothers who breastfeed also eat low-carbohydrate diets or exercise five times a week, it would be difficult to determine whether distinct health outcomes were attributable to breastfeeding or to behavior—eating or exercise habits—associated with breastfeeding. Not surprisingly, the more thoroughly studies eliminate these confounding variables, the less impact breastfeeding seems to have.

What researchers call "selection bias," or the possibility that different types of people self-select into different behavioral groups and that their preexisting dissimilarities are responsible for distinct health outcomes, is a serious problem in infant-feeding research. It is possible that mothers who breastfeed tend to behave differently in a variety of health-promoting ways and that it is this behavior, not breastfeeding per se, that is responsible for better health. University of Chicago political scientist Eric Oliver asks a similar question about obesity. In survey data on the health behavior of middle and high school students, he found tooth brushing to be the best predictor of obesity. Dismissing the notion that tooth brushing plays a direct role in children's weight, Oliver argues that it is nonetheless a good indicator of homes in which health and hygiene are priorities, of households where children eat healthier foods and engage in fewer sedentary activities.[1] People who brush their teeth regularly, in other words, undertake multiple health-enhancing behaviors. Women who breastfeed may distinguish themselves similarly. They may talk to and reason with their children in ways that promote intellectual development. They may decrease children's weight problems by encouraging exercise and balanced diets. They may reduce infection by maintaining clean homes and keeping their children from virus-laden places, such as grocery stores at 5 p.m. or shopping malls on the weekend. Hand washing is now considered so important in checking the transmission of viruses and infections that liquid sanitizer dispensers line the corridors of many hospitals. Mothers who wash their hands frequently and have their children do the same could be diminishing exposure to germs in significant ways. Given the widespread belief that breastfeeding is healthier, women who choose to breastfeed might well be the same mothers who consistently go the extra mile to ward off sickness. This is not to say that formula-feeding mothers do not care about their children. But *on average*, if women who breastfeed are more preoccupied with health, their behavior could go a long way toward explaining any differences between breastfed and formula-fed babies.

Moreover, in careful research, when breastfed babies are found to be healthier, they are only modestly so, and confounding and selection bias are of particular concern in studies where the differences are small. Consistency of result does not solve this problem. There is an old joke about a business that loses money on everything it sells but hopes to make it up in volume. Likewise, if one study with critical methodological flaws is not convincing, one hundred or one thousand studies with the same weaknesses are no more compelling. Meta-analyses, literature reviews, and commentaries that do not seriously take into account confounding and bias are also unreliable. As the number of years between breastfeeding and the measured health outcome grows, so too does the list of possibly influential factors, which means that the challenge of isolating cause and effect is magnified when trying to evaluate long-term benefits. Those who claim that bottle-fed babies are more likely to be obese or to suffer from diabetes as adults face the nearly insurmountable task of establishing a link between infant feeding and the onset of disease several years or decades later.

So when studies find a correlation between breastfeeding and better health, this does not mean that breastfeeding *causes* better health; the advantages might well come from the overall health behavior of women who choose to initiate or continue breastfeeding, routines that could be adopted by bottle-feeding mothers. It might be that breastfeeding is part of a package of ostensibly health-promoting behaviors, any one of which is insignificant on its own, and that the decision to breastfeed represents an approach to parenting that itself has a positive impact on children's health. Current research, therefore, justifies neither the widespread belief that breastfeeding has extensive advantages nor the NBAC's claim that formula feeding is dangerous. In fact, a great deal of evidence suggests that the choice between breast- and bottle-feeding has little impact on most babies in the United States.

Unavoidable Risks

Every action has risks and benefits, costs and savings, and breastfeeding and bottle-feeding are no different. The problem is that most people don't understand this, and when strong emotions are involved, people tend to become more confused. They focus on worst-case scenarios (what if my child is kidnapped from the backyard?) instead of probability (how likely is it that someone will walk into my backyard and take my child?). They forget that risks need to be considered in terms of other risks, and they lose sight of the inevitable trade-offs that accompany any risk-reducing behavior (if I drive my car instead of flying in an airplane, I'm more likely to die in a car crash). Like most breastfeeding promotion, the NBAC neglected to mention the risks and trade-offs of breastfeeding. For example, breast milk contains environmental contaminants. Despite the fact that most lactating mothers have detectable and at times highly elevated levels of these environmental agents in their milk, breastfeeding advocates and even environmental activists have been reluctant to emphasize this concern for fear of discouraging women from breastfeeding. Conventional risk assessment methods, based on adult body weights and food consumption data, do not consider the ways in which infants and children are uniquely susceptible to chemical exposures via their mothers' milk. Nor do studies that isolate single contaminants effectively measure environmental risk. Furthermore, extensive research indicates that babies in homes where mothers are psychologically depressed or economically stressed are at risk for a variety of developmental and health disorders. For women who find the demands of breastfeeding overwhelming or who cannot manage to breastfeed on the job, formula-feeding might well be the less risky way to feed their babies. The point here is not that environmental contaminants or threats to women's emotional well-being make breastfeeding *necessarily* dangerous. It is rather that both breastfeeding and formula-feeding have costs, or risks, and that women and their families need to make choices about which risks they can tolerate.

Risks are ubiquitous, but we only pay attention to some of them. Certain cars, for example, have better safety records than others. The air in congested cities and suburbs is more highly polluted and raises the risk of asthma and other illnesses. Yet parents are not the targets of public health campaigns like the NBAC that implore them to move to less populated areas or to trade their SUVs for safer minivans. A sustained effort by interest groups, doctors, and the government to move babies from urban areas in order to reduce the risk of asthma likely would be met with skepticism. Parents would discuss trade-offs, or costs and benefits, and most probably would elect to stay in their relatively polluted neighborhoods. Riding in cars can be deadly, and although safety seats provide some protection, parents who drive with their babies and children routinely put them at risk. Yet it is difficult to imagine a cultivated campaign to keep families out of cars. Should such an effort materialize, it would likely be met with resistance. Few people would say that even the chance of a car accident makes driving too dangerous, and most would judge the costs of not driving to be too high, despite the health risks. Infant feeding also involves trade-offs. Bottle-feeding, like all consumer behavior, contributes to global warming and deforestation, and from an environmental perspective, breastfeeding has advantages over formula-feeding. But breastfeeding also has risks that must be calculated in the feeding decision. Mothers who leave employment temporarily—for example, to be full-time caretakers for their young children—are more likely to struggle financially in old age, and they are at greater risk for poverty in cases of divorce. Yet the perils for women of not sustaining employment are largely ignored while the putative risks of not breastfeeding (or of sending young children to day care) are well publicized. Again, the lesson here is not that all families should stop driving and move to the country, or that no mother should take time from work to be with her babies or children. Rather, it is to demonstrate that we make risky decisions every day without knowing it, and that we pay comparatively more attention to risks that require short- and long-term sacrifices from mothers.

The Costs of Breastfeeding

Breastfeeding is not free. It is often described that way, however, because maternal labor is understood to be natural and therefore without cost. So while the rhetoric of the NBAC was hyperbolic and observers were likely to recognize the obvious exaggerations in the campaign's imagery, it all made sense in a culture that expects mothers to protect their children from any conceivable threat. In an era when Americans seem convinced that they can eliminate just about any risk, a cultural message has developed that mothers not only must shield their children from immediate threats but also must be experts in everything their children might encounter. Mothers are held uniquely responsible for predicting and preventing any circumstance that might interfere with their children's putatively normal development, and they are exhorted to optimize every dimension of their children's lives, beginning with the womb. They are told by multiple authorities to monitor their bodies in order to optimize "pre-conception," conception, pregnancy, and childbirth, and they are advised that no risk to a child is too small to eliminate and no cost too high to bear in the effort.

This moral code, an ethic of "total motherhood," is frequently cast as a trade-off between what babies and children need versus what mothers might like. No doubt passion for breastfeeding and antipathy for infant formula are rooted in concern about babies. But they also derive from the taken-for-granted belief that a moral mother will subjugate herself completely to a socially defined, all-inclusive notion of the needs of children. When mothers have only *wants*, such as a sense of bodily, emotional, and psychological autonomy, but children have only *needs*, such as an environment in which anything less than optimal is framed as perilous, then good mothers themselves have no needs, repress their wants, and behave in ways that reduce even minuscule or poorly understood risks to their children, regardless of the cost to themselves. Under total motherhood, mothers disappear as women and as individuals. Nowhere is this more clear than in the NBAC's exclusive emphasis on babies, in its choice *not* to address breastfeeding's putative health advantages for mothers, a discussion that likely would have made its case more persuasive. The campaign fused total motherhood and widespread concern about risk with the result that the maternal responsibility to protect babies from the dangers associated with bottle-feeding became a moral imperative.

What is more, the NBAC treated the reasons women might choose not to breastfeed as obstacles to be overcome rather than as trade-offs or costs to be weighed against the benefits attributed to breastfeeding. According to the Ad Council's "Breastfeeding Awareness" Website, women "accept that breast-feeding is the 'best' option—and are generally aware of many specific advantages, but their fears and doubts about their ability and perceived inconvenience often outweigh for them what are perceived as the 'added benefits' of breastfeeding."[2] While promoting the campaign, Surgeon General Richard Carmona told a New York radio station that "very few situations" should "prevent a mom from breastfeeding."[3] In the rhetoric of the NBAC, women's needs—to work, to control their bodies, or to sustain an identity independent of their children—become luxuries that mothers who care about their babies can and should forego. The campaign tried explicitly to connect with African American and working-class women, whose breastfeeding rates are well below those of white and Hispanic women. Outreach included community projects in such cities as Birmingham, San Juan, Baltimore, and Knoxville, inclusion of black actors and soul and country music in public service announcements, and posters and pamphlets that contained photos designed to attract the target audiences. But the NBAC's approach, which essentially treated cultural reasons for not breastfeeding as irrational and workplace obstacles as every mother's personal responsibility to surmount, did not take seriously the costs of breastfeeding for black and lower-income women. Like total motherhood, the message of the campaign was decidedly white and middle-class.

Trade-offs do not disappear when the science is more compelling. Strong evidence exists for the NBAC's claim that breastfeeding reduces the risk of gastrointestinal infection. Breast milk carries antimicrobial proteins, and once babies ingest the milk, these proteins line the gut and combat various bacteria in the GI tract, a process that scientists can observe. But does this evidence justify the NBAC's message? According to one of the most widely respected breastfeeding studies, one in twenty-five bottle-fed babies will have an additional GI infection compared with the same number of breast-fed babies. Is this risk great enough to offset the cost of breastfeeding for a mother who prefers to bottle-feed? Is reducing the risk of an additional bout of diarrhea or vomiting worth the price for women who otherwise would choose, for personal, cultural, or other reasons, not to breastfeed? Are there similar health risks, including those associated with driving, that we ignore every day because we deem the price tag too high? Do we believe that risks to babies and children must be eliminated at any expense, or only if the costs of eliminating these risks can be paid by mothers? The evidence for most of breastfeeding's benefits is weak. But even when it is persuasive, it does not *necessarily* dictate that babies should be breastfed.

Women choose to breastfeed for various reasons. They find breastfeeding more convenient than bottle-feeding; they do not want to support formula manufacturers; they believe, for religious or cultural reasons, that mothers have a unique obligation to their babies, which includes breastfeeding; they want to shrink their carbon footprint and help the environment by reducing formula production. These are all legitimate motivations, but they should not be cloaked in language about the medical dangers of infant formula. If, in the future, science demonstrates that breastfeeding has serious health advantages, then public health officials, women, and their families will have to determine whether the benefits of breastfeeding override its costs. In the meantime, in the overwhelming majority of cases, either breastfeeding or formula-feeding is a healthy option, and this, not the notion that infant formula is dangerous, is what the government should be telling mothers.

NOTES

1. Eric Oliver, *Fat Politics: The Real Story Behind America's Obesity Epidemic* (New York: Oxford University Press, 2006), 165.

2. That Website is now defunct. For a similar message, see the U.S. Department of Health and Human Services' site on breastfeeding at http://www.womenshealth.gov/breastfeeding/.

3. Richard Carmona, "Radio Interviews with Surgeon General Richard H. Carmona," U.S. Department of Health and Human Services, http://www.womenshealth.gov/archive/breastfeeding/programs/nbc/interviews/2.cfm.

Part III —

Making Health and Disease

8

Pharmaceutical Propaganda

CARL ELLIOTT

Several years ago, I was sitting in my office at the University of Minnesota, trying to avoid work, when I got an unusual phone call.[1] It came from an international advertising agency. The woman on the phone said she had read my book, *Better than Well*, and wondered if I would talk about it at a meeting in Boston. I had no idea what to make of her invitation. It was hard for me to imagine why anyone in an advertising agency would want to hear about my book, which was not exactly enthusiastic about the marketing business. Besides, this company did not even seem to market drugs. They advertised consumer products like cars, bourbon whiskey, and golf balls. Out of curiosity, I agreed to go.

The meeting was for the company's "strategic planners," who had been flown to Boston from various international locations. Strategic planners, I learned, are hip young people who dress in black and wear small, stylish glasses. In the advertising world, their job description appears to fall somewhere between "ethnographer" and "evil genius." Unlike "the creatives," who were not present at the meeting but were often invoked, like mysterious spirits, strategic planners do not actually create ads. They are the intellectuals behind the operation. It is part of their job to hit the streets, sniff the air, and figure out what can be exploited for capitalism. The strategic planners had gathered in Boston to brainstorm about their various marketing campaigns, one of which concerned a new Volkswagen.

The Volkswagen campaign was tricky. Volkswagen was producing a luxury car called the Phaeton, which it planned to price at over $70,000. Volkswagen envisioned the Phaeton as an elite, high-end competitor to Jaguar, BMW, and Mercedes. For the strategic planners, the problem with the Phaeton was the Volkswagen brand. Volkswagens are not exactly branded for luxury. If anything, they are branded with a kind of hip nostalgia for the 1960s' counterculture. So the strategic planners had a dilemma. To sell a luxury car like the Phaeton, they had to reach luxury car buyers. But they did not want to alienate the Volkswagen brand loyalists. How do you sell luxury Volkswagens without looking like a sellout to all those guys in denim jackets and gray ponytails, who associate Volkswagens with the smell of weed and the sound of the Grateful Dead?

After months of research, the strategic planners had constructed a detailed plan. To sell luxury Volkswagens, they believed, you need to find a particular kind of customer. Ideally, these customers are creative, environmentally sensitive liberals who are concerned about social justice. They are the sort of people who read the *New York Times*, listen to National Public Radio, and shop at Whole Foods. They spend a lot of time in coffee shops and bookstores, and they are closely involved with their neighborhood organizations and their children's schools. And of course, they have stock portfolios impressive enough for them to drop $70,000 on a luxury car.

Unfortunately, however, there is a problem with this particular psychographic. They are deeply cynical about advertising. Only rarely do they watch television, and when they do, they filter out all the ads with TiVos. So how do you market to them? Here is where I began to grasp the dark allure of strategic planning. The planners were going to find out what left-wing charities their customers favored, where their kids went to school, and what neighborhood organizations they were involved in. Then they planned to donate money to those groups and make sure everyone knew about it, as a way to generate word-of-mouth buzz. My host at the meeting, a former literature professor who now worked as a "cultural strategist" for the company, was practically rubbing his hands with delight. He kept leaning over to me and whispering things like, "So what would Marx think about this one, eh?" and "Talk about seizing the means of production!"

As ingenious as the plan was, it appears to have backfired spectacularly. When the Phaeton was introduced to the United States, the *New York Times* featured an article on the car headlined, "A People's Car for Wealthy People."[2] In 2004, only 1,433 cars were sold, and when sales dropped the next year to a mere 820, Volkswagen announced that the Phaeton would be discontinued. (It was later reintroduced.) It is hard to know whether these disappointing sales were a result of an ill-conceived marketing campaign, or if the problem was the Phaeton itself. However, the difficulty marketing the Phaeton is symptomatic of a deeper predicament facing any advertising agency today. How do you market a product to customers who are thoroughly contemptuous of marketing?

Drug marketers have faced this problem for years. Prescription drugs are bought and sold as market commodities, but nobody is entirely comfortable thinking of them as consumer goods. Prescribing decisions are supposed to be made on the basis of scientific evidence, not whim or preference; the decision-makers are highly educated professionals who are supposed to put the patient's interests first; and the stakes involved in a single prescription can be alarmingly high. Few of us are unreservedly enthusiastic about inserting pharmaceutical sales into the machinery of consumer capitalism, at least when our own health is on the line. It would be as if the NASA engineers who decide which materials to use for the space shuttle made their decisions based on which company had produced the most ironic television ads.

For the psychic comfort of everyone involved, drug marketing needs to be disguised. Developing this disguise is the job of public relations. The public relations specialist does not market a product so much as manipulate conditions in such a way that more of the product is sold. The manipulation must be accomplished subtly and carefully, without calling too much attention to itself, for if the disguise falls off, the campaign will fail. Yet the covert nature of public relations makes it feel especially fraught. You organize a charity event, but your real purpose is to publicize a drug. You pitch a news story, but your real aim is to market a car. Gradually, you begin to see all the makings of ordinary life as potential marketing devices. This kind of marketing is uncomfortable in a creepy new way. News, conversation, friendship, humanitarian aid: virtually anything can be used as a sales instrument, which is effective only as long as nobody realizes that a product is being sold.

Shortly after my Boston meeting, I came across a book by Al and Laura Ries called *The Fall of Advertising and the Rise of PR*.[3] Ries, a former ad man, lists a string of successful companies, from Starbucks and The Body Shop to Amazon and Intel, which built their brands almost entirely without advertising. "We have seen the future of marketing," Ries said in a 2004 lecture in New York. "The future of marketing is Botox."[4] The audience laughed, but Ries was not joking. When Allergan introduced Botox in 1993, Ries said, the drug generated $25 million in sales. Yet by 2001, Botox was generating $300 million in sales. How did Allergan manage an elevenfold increase in sales in only eight years? "No advertising, no advertising, no advertising, no direct mail," Ries said. "No nothing but PR."

Suppose you were offered a choice, says Ries. A magazine will give you a free advertisement, or they will run your story as an article. "How many companies would prefer an ad to an article?" Ries asks. "No one. Advertising has no credibility."[5] But many people still believe what they read in magazines. It is this credibility that public relations exploits. The public relations expert is always asking himself: how do I take the credibility of a trusted authority and use it for my own purposes?

A pharmaceutical public relations strategy which has been around since the 1950s, but which really picked up steam in the 1990s, is to sell a treatment by selling a disease. To sell Prilosec, you have to sell acid reflux; to sell Lotronex, you have to sell irritable bowel syndrome; to sell Viagra, you have to sell erectile dysfunction; to sell Adderall, you have to sell ADHD. You market a treatment by convincing doctors and patients to diagnose the illness that your drug or procedure treats.

What kind of authority can you use to sell a disease? A useful source is patient advocacy groups. One early example is the Human Growth Foundation, a nonprofit charity based in Virginia.[6] Its aim is to raise awareness about growth disorders. In the early 1990s, the foundation was training gym teachers to measure schoolchildren using special devices and to plot their growth on a growth chart. If a child fell in the bottom fifth percentile for height, the foundation would send the child's parents a letter telling them to get in touch with the foundation or with a doctor. But when outsiders started to look more closely at the foundation, they discovered that its financial backers were Genentech and Eli Lilly, which both manufacture synthetic human growth hormone. Synthetic human growth hormone is the treatment for growth hormone deficiency. It was also approved and marketed later on even for short children without growth hormone deficiency.

In the 1990s, a patient advocacy group backed by a pharmaceutical company was seen as scandalous. Today, it is the norm.[7] For example, CHADD, the attention deficit disorder charity, is funded by the makers of stimulant drugs; the Society for Women's Health Research is funded by Eli Lilly, the maker of Sarafem; and the anxiety support group, Freedom from Fear, is funded by GlaxoSmithKline, the maker of Paxil, a treatment for social anxiety disorder. Disease awareness campaigns are a big part of this kind of marketing, especially diseases with blurry boundaries that can be expanded. The Campaign for America's Mental Health is funded by antidepressant makers; Screening for Mental Health, Inc. is funded by the makers of Prozac and Zoloft; and a depression in college awareness campaign is funded by Wyeth, which makes the antidepressant Effexor. In fact, according to the president of the National Patient Advocate Foundation, there is not a single advocacy group in the country that does not get some funding from the pharmaceutical industry.[8]

The rising power of patients as drug marketers has come at a time when the authority and prestige of physicians has declined. As physicians began to see themselves more and more as businesspeople in the 1980s and '90s, their independent authority as professionals waned in the eyes of patients. If physicians are trying to sell you something, you can no longer simply assume they have your best interests at heart. Patients, on the other hand, stand in a different position. At least on the surface, patients do not have any obvious financial interest in marketing a drug. Nor do they have deep medical knowledge. Their authority comes from another place—not scientific training or clinical expertise, but firsthand experience of an illness and its treatment. In public relations, their role is to front a marketing campaign and give it a sympathetic human face.

In 2001, for instance, the pharmaceutical companies Pfizer and Eisai were promoting Aricept, a drug intended to slow the progression of Alzheimer's disease. Because Alzheimer's is diagnosed solely by the patient's symptoms (no laboratory or imaging tests are available), it was a promising candidate for a "disease awareness" campaign. In concert with the Alzheimer's Association, a Chicago-based patient group, Pfizer and Eisai hired two public relations companies to publicize the disease—Hill and Knowlton, the international PR giant, and TBWA/Health, a smaller company specializing in healthcare communications. To drive home the message that Alzheimer's was unfairly stigmatized, this public relations team orchestrated a remarkably effective series of media events.

First, they produced a public service announcement (PSA) with the Alzheimer's Association, featuring clips of Rita Hayworth, who died with Alzheimer's in 1987. A PSA is a segment that television and radio stations run between regular programs, like advertisements, which are intended to change public attitudes about an issue. (Perhaps the most famous PSA is the "This is your brain on drugs" spots sponsored by the Partnership for a Drug-Free America in the 1980s.) Most PSAs concern issues around health or safety: just say no to drugs; don't drive drunk; send money to feed starving children in Africa. Although some PSAs are sponsored by nonprofit groups, many are backed by corporations. A pharmaceutical industry–backed PSA might ask people to get a flu shot, have their cholesterol checked, or undergo screening for Alzheimer's disease. One great advantage of PSAs is their low cost of production, often less than $50,000 for television and under $20,000 for a radio spot. And unlike advertisements, which may cost millions to place on television, PSAs are broadcast for free. They are considered a non-commercial civic good, like children's shows or community broadcasting.

The PR agencies promoting Aricept recruited Rita Hayworth's daughter to unveil their PSA at the World Alzheimer's Congress. Then they went a step further. In a publicity tactic worthy of a postmodern cultural theorist, the agencies filmed a video news release (VNR) of the unveiling of their own

PSA. A VNR is a simulated television news story designed to be indistinguishable from ordinary television news. Its purpose is to generate publicity for an idea or a product, usually with the aim of selling it. Critics call VNRs "fake news," but according to public relations specialists, they are simply the television equivalent of a press release. Television stations began using VNRs more widely in the 1980s, when local budgets began to drop and stations needed an inexpensive way to fill airtime. Over time, VNRs became a popular way for pharmaceutical companies to generate coverage of new drugs. Most pharmaceutical VNRs hook the segment to an actual event, such as the approval of the drug by the FDA. The brilliance of the Aricept VNR is that it was hooked to the unveiling of a PSA that the agencies themselves had produced, thus generating both a fake news event and fake news coverage of the event.

The PR campaign returned impressive results. The Rita Hayworth PSA ran 12,000 times on 257 stations. Several hundred reporters came to the World Alzheimer's Congress, many of them from international news organizations. President Clinton announced a $50 million NIH funding package for research on Alzheimer's disease, and *Time* magazine ran a cover story. In only ten days, the campaign recorded over 800 million media impressions—more than the Alzheimer's Association usually gets in an entire year. The public relations team even persuaded a producer for the television show *ER* to write Aricept into a show that featured Alan Alda as a patient with early-stage Alzheimer's. So effective was the campaign that it was awarded two "Recognizing Excellence" awards for "raising awareness about a previously disregarded disease."[9]

As useful as patients can be as publicity tools, however, physicians are more effective at one very important task: persuading other physicians to prescribe a given drug. The semi-official terms for these influential physicians is "thought leaders" or "Key Opinion Leaders" (KOLs). KOLs are the experts that a company pays to be consultants, advisory board members, or speakers. Many KOLs speak on behalf of an industry sponsor at conferences, symposia, dinner lectures, and grand rounds presentations. Good KOLs are highly valued; companies can buy books, software packages, and expert consultation on how best to identify and recruit them. One pamphlet, which can be downloaded from the Internet for $5,500, advises pharmaceutical companies to ask the questions, "Will the KOL be cost-effective, influence the market, and agree to speak at conferences on your agreed agenda?"[10]

A more controversial tactic is to hire KOLs to "author" journal articles produced by ghostwriters at medical communications agencies. The agency will hire ghostwriters to write articles, approach academic physicians to attach their names to the articles, and then submit them to medical journals. Medical ghostwriting is not new, but it was once thought to be rare. Recent signs suggest it is more widespread than most observers once suspected. For instance, when Fen-Phen was linked to valvular heart disease and primary pulmonary hypertension in the mid-1990s, litigation revealed a number of ghostwritten articles funded by Wyeth, its manufacturer, and produced by the medical communications company Excerpta Medica. Several years later, it was discovered that Wyeth also produced ghostwritten articles about Premarin, its hormone replacement therapy, even after it was linked to an increased risk of heart disease. GlaxoSmithKline promoted its antidepressant Paxil through a novel ghostwriting program aimed at recruiting physicians to "author" case studies. It was called Case Study Publications for Peer Review, which the company shortened to the acronym, CASPPER.[11]

After Vioxx, the anti-inflammatory drug, was pulled from the market after being linked to heart disease, litigation turned up not merely ghostwritten articles, but entire ghostwritten journals. In Australia, Merck contracted with a subsidiary of the scientific publisher Elsevier to produce a publication titled *Australasian Journal of Bone and Joint Medicine*. The publication looked much like a legitimate journal, complete with a masthead of prominent academic advisors. But in fact, it was a marketing tool for Merck products. Of the twenty-nine articles in the second issue of the journal, nine were related to Vioxx, and twelve were connected to Fosamax, an osteoporosis drug also produced by Merck. Unsurprisingly, the articles all reached positive conclusions about Merck products, and none disclosed the funding source. Excerpta Medica, the Elsevier-owned medical communications agency that produced the journal, also produced fake journals such as the *Australasian Journal of General Practice*, the *Australasian Journal of Neurology*, the *Australasian Journal of Cardiology*, the *Australasian Journal of Clinical Pharmacy*, and the *Australasian Journal of Cardiovascular Medicine*.[12]

No one really knows how much of the medical literature is ghostwritten, but a hint emerged in a 2003 study in the *British Journal of Psychiatry* (*BJP*).[13] A lawsuit brought against Pfizer in 1999 had turned up documents produced by a medical communications company called Current Medical Directions, which was responsible for a publication strategy for Pfizer's antidepressant, Zoloft. These documents listed all the Zoloft studies that Current Medical Directions was preparing for publication in 1999.

The authors of the *BJP* article, David Healy and Dinah Cattell, decided to track down the articles on Zoloft that Current Medical Directions had been working on in 1999 and see what had happened to them. They picked three years (1998, 1999, and 2000) and searched the medical literature for all articles published on Zoloft during that time. They found that the agency-prepared articles outnumbered the articles written in the traditional way, were published in more prestigious journals, and had citation rates over five times that of traditionally authored articles. The ghosted articles also painted a much happier profile of Zoloft than did the traditionally authored articles. For example, the articles prepared by Current Medical Directions on pediatric psychopharmacology failed to mention five of the six children taking Zoloft who took action toward committing suicide.

The academic physicians who sign on to these articles are not merely useful as "authors" and speakers. They can also be useful in helping the drug industry get past regulatory barriers. This point was explained quite frankly over thirty years ago in a book called *The Regulation Games*.[14] In a section titled "Co-opt the Experts," the authors note that academics often have a significant influence on regulatory policy, and that a company needs to get them on board if it expects be successful. The authors advise companies to identify the relevant academic experts, hire them as consultants or advisors, give them research grants, and convince them that they are giving them the money because the company needs their expertise. The company has to finesse this, say the authors, because academics must not recognize that they have lost their objectivity.

One example of the importance of such relationships can be seen in the debate over whether the SSRI antidepressants increase the risk of suicide. For the better part of the past twenty years there has been an active controversy over whether the FDA should require antidepressant makers to include a "black box" warning label on antidepressants, warning clinicians of the risk of suicidal ideation. In 2004, the FDA decided to require a black box label when these medications are prescribed to children. But that requirement was a departure from the decision arrived at by the FDA thirteen years earlier. In September 1991, the FDA panel that looked at antidepressants and suicide had a very different composition, and it arrived at a very different conclusion. Five of the ten advisory committee members in 1991 had financial relationships with manufacturers of antidepressants. Of six consultants to the committee, three had financial relationships with antidepressant manufacturers. One committee member had received over $1.4 million from Eli Lilly, the maker of Prozac. After one day of testimony, the advisory committee decided that there was no link between antidepressants and suicide, and that no black box warning was needed.[15]

The transcripts of that meeting say, "All committee members may participate in the meeting without the risk of any conflict of interest." This is not unusual. For years the FDA has granted waivers to advisory committee members with financial relationships to the pharmaceutical industry, claiming that such relationships are so ubiquitous that it is impossible to identify academics with the relevant expertise who have not worked with industry. A recent survey found that over half of all FDA experts had financial ties to the industries whose drugs they were regulating. In meetings where general issues were being discussed, over 90 percent had financial conflicts.[16]

Compromised regulators, greedy physicians, ghosted journal articles, fake news reports—it all seems pretty difficult to defend, at least on ethical grounds. Are bioethicists working furiously to root out pharmaceutical money from the academy? Not exactly. By the early 2000s, it had become clear that the field of bioethics has many industry connections of its own.[17] Many bioethicists work for industry as private consultants. Others serve on "ethics advisory boards" for pharmaceutical or biotechnology companies. A few hold industry-funded chairs. Some of the best-known bioethics centers support themselves with donations and grants from industry, such as The Hastings Center and the Center for Bioethics at the University of Pennsylvania. In the late 1990s, the American Medical Association even started an initiative to educate doctors about the ethics of industry gifts, yet it funded the initiative with nearly $600,000 in industry gifts.

The cleverest use of bioethics to support a public relations campaign was devised by a small PR firm called Belsito and Company on behalf of Xigris, a drug produced by Eli Lilly for the treatment of sepsis.[18] (Sepsis is an infection of the blood that can threaten the lives of hospitalized patients.) When Lilly launched Xigris in 2001, it hoped that the drug would be a blockbuster. Prozac had recently lost its patent protection, and the company needed a replacement. But Xigris did not take off. One reason may have been that Xigris was no better than older treatments for sepsis. The main reason, however, was its cost. Standard treatments for sepsis usually cost less than $50 per day, while Xigris cost a whopping $6,800 per treatment. So Belsito designed a public relations campaign called "The Ethics, the Urgency and the Potential," the premise being that it is unethical to deny Xigris to patients merely because of its expense. To reinforce the point, Lilly funded a $1.8 million project called the "Values, Ethics & Rationing in Critical Care Task Force" (VERICC) in which bioethicists and physicians from various American medical schools examined the ethics of rationing certain drugs and services. "Robert Lieberman is lucky to be alive," reported a New York station, in a news segment on the VERICC task force. "He was on a ventilator near death when he got a new biotech drug called Xigris that probably saved his life."

Apparently, bioethics is an excellent vehicle for selling drugs. When the Xigris campaign was finished, the Council of Public Relations Firms highlighted the VERICC task force as a successful case study, pointing out that VERICC was covered by sixty media outlets, attracted over 132 million viewers, and was covered by *The Wall Street Journal*, National Public Radio, ABC World News Tonight, *The Toronto Star*, and *The Boston Globe*. By early 2004, Xigris sales were up 36 percent.

The father of American public relations, Edward Bernays, described his vision of public relations in his 1928 book, *Propaganda*. The public relations counsel should aspire to be a detached professional, Bernays argued, one of the "invisible governors" at the top who coolly observe and manipulate the receptive, unthinking masses. "It is they who pull the wires which control the public mind," wrote Bernays, "who harness old social forces and contrive new ways to bind and guide the world."[19] The phrase "invisible governors" was prophetic. Today the average American probably could not name a single public relations company or even say what they do, yet the techniques of public relations permeate the culture in a way that is hard to exaggerate. We live in a political landscape filled with lobby groups and public opinion pollsters. The corporate world is dominated by multinational public relations companies such as Weber Shandwick, Hill and Knowlton, Ketchum, and Burson-Marsteller. No company, university, or government body of any size is without a communications office, whose job it is to protect the interests and reputation of its employer. The elitist vision of Bernays may have gone out of fashion, but marketers and politicians have embraced the tactics he developed. Unlike many traditional marketers, however, who must dance frantically in the spotlight to sell their products, the public relations expert watches silently from the wings.

When academics look at the ethical issues surrounding the pharmaceutical industry, they generally frame the problem as a "conflict of interest," which can be solved by identifying and managing the conflicts that arise for doctors, authors, or researchers. Yet "conflict of interest" does not really describe the full extent of the problem presented by public relations. "Conflict of interest" suggests that the basic problem is with individuals, whose duties may be compromised by their financial interests. A better term would be "corruption," which suggests that this is a problem for social institutions. The problem with "video news releases" is that they undermine the real news.

The problem with ghostwritten journal articles is that they undermine legitimate journal articles. The problem with industry-funded bioethics is that it undermines the notion that academics are free of vested interests in the topics that they teach. This kind of undermining is the real problem—not only the personal conflicts of individuals, but the undermining of social institutions that depend on trust. Institutions are difficult to build, but they can be surprisingly easy to destroy. Once trust in an institution is lost, it is very hard to recover.

NOTES

1. This chapter is adapted from Carl Elliott, *White Coat, Black Hat: Adventures on the Dark Side of Medicine* (Boston: Beacon Press, 2010).

2. James G. Cobb, "2004 Volkswagen Phaeton V-8: A People's Car for Wealthy People," *New York Times*, January 25, 2004, http://www.nytimes.com/2004/01/25/automobiles/25auto.html?pagewanted=all.

3. Al Ries and Laura Ries, *The Fall of Advertising and the Rise of PR* (New York: HarperBusiness, 2002).

4. "Marketing in the Post-Advertising Era—Edelman Seminar July 11, 2002," Edelman, http://www.edelman.com/events/Post-Advertising/transcript_w.asp?speed=56.

5. Ries and Ries, *The Fall of Advertising*, 90.

6. See Ralph T. King, Jr., "Charity Tactic by Genentech Stirs Questions," *Wall Street Journal*, Aug 10, 1994, B1.

7. See Thomas Ginsberg, "Donations Tie Drug Firms and Nonprofits," *Philadelphia Inquirer*, May 28, 2006, http:/8.

8. Jim Drinkard, "Drugmakers Go Furthest to Sway Congress," USA Today, April 25, 2005, http://www.usatoday.com/money/industries/health/drugs/2005-04-25-drug-lobby-cover_x.htm.

9. "Alzheimer's Campaign Peaks Public and Media Interest," *PR News* 57, no. 20 (May 21, 2001): 1.

10. Best Practices, LLC, "Optimizing Key Opinion Leader Relationships: Best Practices in KOL Management," http://www3.best-in-class.com/bestp/domrep.nsf/Content/1682B4305DAC5CE88525756A0037C5E2!OpenDocument.

11. Matthew Perrone, "Glaxo Used Ghostwriting to Promote Paxil," *Boston Globe*, August 20, 2009, http://www.boston.com/news/health/articles/2009/08/20/glaxosmithkline_used_ghostwriting_to_promote_paxil/.

12. Bob Grant, "Elsevier Published Six Fake Journals," *The Scientist.com*, May 7, 2009, http://www.the-scientist.com/templates/trackable/display/blog.jsp?type=blog&o_url=blog/display/55679&id=55679. See also Grant's "Merck Published Fake Journal," *The Scientist.com*, April 30, 2009, http://www.the-scientist.com/blog/display/55671/.

13. David Healy and Dinah Cattell, "Interface between Authorship, Industry and Science in the Domain of Therapeutics," *British Journal of Psychiatry*, 183 (July 2003): 22–23.

14. Bruce M. Owen and Ronald Braeutigam, *The Regulation Games: Strategic Use of the Administrative Process* (Cambridge, MA: Ballinger Publishing, 1978), 7.

15. See Joseph Glenmullen, *Prozac Backlash: Overcoming the Dangers of Prozac, Zoloft, Paxil, and Other Antidepressants with Safe, Effective Alternatives* (New York: Simon & Schuster, 2001), 156–57.

16. Dennis Cauchon, "FDA Advisers Tied to Industry," *USA Today,* September 25, 2000, 1A.

17. See Sheryl Gay Stolberg, "Bioethicists Find Themselves the Ones Being Scrutinized," *New York Times,* August 2, 2001, http://www.nytimes.com/2001/08/02/us/bioethicists-find-themselves-the-ones-being-scrutinized.html. See also my "Pharma Buys a Conscience," *The American Prospect* 12, no. 2 (September 23, 2001): 16–20.

18. Antonio Regalado, "To Sell Pricey Drug, Lilly Fuels a Debate over Rationing," *Wall Street Journal,* September 18, 2003, A1. See also my own, "Not-So-Public Relations," *Slate.com,* December 15, 2003, http://slate.msn.com/id/2092442/.

19. Edward Bernays, *Propaganda* (Brooklyn, NY: Ig Publishing, 2005), 17.

9

The Strangely Passive-Aggressive History of Passive-Aggressive Personality Disorder

CHRISTOPHER LANE

When psychiatric terms such as "bipolar" and "passive-aggressive" migrate into popular culture and assume everyday meaning, there are several effects that deserve comment and analysis. First, as Georges Canguilhem and others have observed, the boundaries between the normal and the pathological begin to blur. Normality—already a vague, tendentious category—becomes an abstract ideal into which fewer and fewer people squeeze.[1] And what we formally and informally consider pathological behavior expands exponentially, in a process Peter D. Kramer once dubbed "diagnostic bracket creep."[2]

These changes are not merely conceptual. There are tangible outcomes too, such as those borne out of the pharmaceutical industry's vested interest in turning ordinary behaviors into treatable conditions. The 1999 "public awareness" campaign "Imagine Being Allergic to People," which cost GlaxoSmithKline more than $92 million in that year alone, is a good example of this because it encouraged mental health professionals and the general public to redefine shyness as a symptom of social anxiety disorder.[3] One decade later, when GSK's Paxil was a blockbuster drug earning more than $2 billion annually from national sales alone, social anxiety disorder had become the third most diagnosed mental disorder, behind only depression and alcoholism.[4] Twenty years earlier, by contrast, the disorder did not formally exist.

Just as we need to examine how mental disorders are defined and expanded, so is it crucial to assess how the medicalization of routine behaviors and traits undermines our increasingly embattled and tenuous concept of "mental health." One can chart this development in rapid strokes. In 1968, the *Diagnostic and Statistical Manual of Mental Disorders* cited 180 categories of mental disorders. By 1987, that number had grown to 292 and, by 1994, with the publication of *DSM-IV*, to over 350. In just twenty-six years, that is, the total number of mental disorders that the general population might exhibit almost doubled.

"About half of Americans will meet the criteria for a *DSM-IV* diagnosis sometime in their life,"[5] investigators at Harvard Medical School declared almost casually after updating the last National Comorbidity Survey, completed a decade earlier. By their lights it should not surprise us that in 2002, over 67.5 million people in the United States—nearly a quarter of the population—had taken SSRI medication for depression and anxiety, just two of the 350 disorders now formally recognized.[6] (To offer a snapshot of one more disorder, estimates put the spike in diagnoses of bipolar disorder "in recent years" at 4,000 percent.)[7]

To help explain how such "diagnostic bracket creep" continues to influence American psychiatry, this chapter takes as its test case the *DSM* inclusion and expansion of "passive-aggressive personality disorder." While the *DSM*'s proliferating categories have generated extensive commentary and analysis,[8] little has been written about this particular disorder or the extent to which it has influenced popular culture. My focus is largely historical, tracing the disorder's roots to World War II before charting its rapid development as the psychiatric profession applied it to ever-larger segments of the civilian population. My aim in revisiting this material, most of it unknown to psychiatrists, much less the general public, is to dramatize the American Psychiatric Association's conceptual and practical difficulties in differentiating normal from pathological behavior, not least because its own diagnostic manual has done so much to blur meaningful distinctions between the two.

Like many other psychiatric terms that have captured the public imagination, the label "passive-aggressive" far exceeds its diagnostic purview. It is now widely accepted shorthand for a person with hostility issues. Experts weigh in on its causes while popular Websites encourage the frustrated to rail at manipulative bosses, conniving coworkers, obnoxious neighbors, and delinquent roommates. Sixty years ago, the phrase "passive-aggressive" didn't exist; now, like "bipolar" and "obsessive-compulsive," it is almost ubiquitous. What does this prevalence tell us about the evolution of American psychiatry, including its transformative effect on our thinking?

The history of passive-aggressive personality disorder is one answer, even though that history is in fact as strange and open-ended as the behavior it describes. It dates to a single Technical Bulletin issued by the U.S. Department of War just as World War II was coming to an end. In October 1945, Colonel William C. Menninger voiced concern about soldiers who were shirking duty by willful incompetence. The soldiers weren't openly defiant, he warned, but expressed their aggressiveness "by passive measures, such as pouting, stubbornness, procrastination, inefficiency, and passive obstructionism."[9] Menninger saw their behavior as an "immaturity" reaction to "routine military stress." Given the number of fronts on which the country was fighting at the time, the stress that American servicemen endured doesn't seem "routine." But while it is easy to grasp why the military would want to maximize efficiency, issuing a memo against "pouting" doesn't seem like a viable solution. Adds Cecil Adams on *The Straight Dope*, "If you've ever served in the military during wartime or for that matter read *Catch-22*, you realize that what the brass calls a personality disorder a grunt might call a rational strategy to avoid getting killed."[10]

The term didn't disappear when the war ended. On the contrary, the armed forces found it a useful way of characterizing unwelcome behavior and spent a good deal of energy over the next few years ridiculing those said to exhibit it. The composite sketches they drew of "passive, henpecked Mr. Milquetoast[s]" made them look more like Norman Bates in Alfred Hitchcock's thriller *Psycho* than that of Michael Scott in the TV series *The Office*.[11] "The passive-dependent character is a boy in man's clothes," sneered Lieutenant James R. Hodge in a 1955 edition of the *United States Armed Forces Medical Journal*, as he steered the charge from aggression to over-reliance; "he is the child who never got away from his mother's apron strings." "After he is married, if he ever is . . . he brings his marital squabbles home to Mamma's big bosom and embracing arms."[12] Four more pages of similar invective ensue. Apparently it was simpler for Lieutenant Hodge to scorn his subordinates than view their questioning as sometimes justified. After all, the latter stance played a critical role in later wars such as Vietnam.

What happened next is even more intriguing. Having logged the quirks of servicemen, psychiatrists began applying them virtually unaltered to civilians. As it readied the first edition of the *DSM* for publication in 1952, the American Psychiatric Association (APA) simply copied the relevant phrases from the military memo. With startling unoriginality or passive dependence, it adopted the same practice for many other ailments, making the temporary frustration of the U.S. Department of War the basis for diagnosing lasting pathologies in the population at large.

The *DSM* soon became the bible of mental health, quoted chapter and verse in schools, courts, prisons, insurance companies, and doctors' offices around the world. Psychiatrists today like to portray it as a watertight document based on evidence and hard science. Few of them know or care to admit that its foundation was really a batch of sketchy military memos.

In the 1950s, unit cohesion wasn't the APA's primary concern; it fretted more about disobedience at work and home. So when the organization's first edition of the *DSM* appeared, conflicts in the workplace or family assumed new meaning. Experts could—and did—call them aggressiveness conveyed "by passive measures, such as pouting, stubbornness, procrastination, inefficiency, and passive obstruction."[13]

That such common traits as dithering and petulance could stem from a passive-aggressive personality began to take root in the culture, where the notion blossomed in such related contexts as marriage counseling.[14] By 1966, passive-aggressive personality disorder was a common psychiatric diagnosis, accounting for more than 3 percent of hospitalized patients in public mental institutions and over 9 percent of outpatient clinic patients.[15] Given the open-endedness of the *DSM* criteria, one shudders to think what was really driving these statistics. After all, a diagnosis of "stubbornness" could be made of housewives not modeled on their Stepford counterparts; men rather like Willy Loman, in Arthur Miller's *Death of a Salesman*, could be labeled "inefficient" if they were struggling with their assigned (and frequently undervalued) role.

DSM-I was in fact amazingly careless in describing the behaviors that it deemed pathological, painting them with a very broad brush. If you were diagnosed with an "emotionally unstable personality," it might be because the psychiatrist thought you displayed "fluctuating emotional attitudes" that day. Perhaps you simply changed your mind too often, but the same pathology would also bring you dangerously close to passive-aggressive personality disorder. Meanwhile, the *DSM* applied the term "sociopathic personality disturbance" to those thought "ill in terms of society and of conformity with the prevailing cultural milieu," a phrase with an almost Orwellian sound.[16]

On at least two occasions, however, the APA exercised its own independence, with disastrous consequences. It struck the word "reaction" from most conflicts, instead defining symptoms in terms of "personality." And it viewed these as "pathologic" rather than "psychopathic." If the American military had complained about minor military infractions tied to specific situations, the APA soon broadcast that the businessman or housewife with a "passive-aggressive personality" revealed a pathologic "trait disturbance." Marking a clear deviation from normalcy, their behavior was a syndrome that might recur if left untreated. The APA wasn't simply overdramatizing routine behaviors; it was relabeling them as malfunctions of biology and neurology, the direction in which American psychiatry overall was heading.

After another round of edits in the late 1960s, the same "traits" became "deeply ingrained maladaptive patterns of behavior," which according to *DSM-II* were usually "life-long" and "determined primarily by malfunctioning of the brain."[17] The APA was now close to saying that passive-aggression and all other mental disorders were permanent, even innate, conditions. The manual's second edition also deleted the word "reaction" from all remaining psychiatric categories. As a result, diagnoses such as "schizophrenic reaction," which previously had referred to sporadic psychiatric incidents, rapidly ballooned into full-blown "schizophrenia," even if the person's symptoms were rare and not especially violent.

This bold stroke amounted to a major shift in approach. It changed the very meaning and ontology of illnesses for clinicians and patients and eliminated the dynamism or struggle of the patient's reaction. Illnesses began to define people rather than surfacing as an aspect of their personality, and symptoms weren't just an expression of unease. They were maladaptive problems that psychiatrists must treat and that society in general should fear.

To passive-aggressive personality disorder, in particular, *DSM-II* added two quite ominous sentences that greatly increased the likelihood of misdiagnosis: "This behavior commonly reflects hostility which the individual feels he dare not express openly. Often the behavior is one expression of the patient's resentment at failing to find gratification in a relationship with an individual or institution upon which he is over-dependent."[18] Not only had the *DSM* outlawed pouting; it left those with ungratifying jobs vulnerable to a psychiatric diagnosis too.

While it's difficult to believe these statements could exist in a manual of mental disorders that had global recognition, of greater embarrassment to American psychiatry is that *DSM-III*, appearing in 1980, didn't improve on them but made a bad situation worse. Robert L. Spitzer, chair of its task force on "Nomenclature and Statistics," bragged that the new edition would at last be evidence-based and rule-driven, forming a "classification system that would reflect our current state of knowledge regarding mental disorders."[19] But after several years' discussion, the group—pathologizing at least one of the behaviors that it itself exhibited—thought it sufficient to add "dawdling and 'forgetfulness'" to the disorder's possible symptoms.[20] They must have believed that these additions paved the way for the profession's newfound scientific direction.

To an extent far greater than its contributors and editors care to admit, *DSM-III* is a deeply flawed and embarrassing document. It advises psychiatrists that "schizoid personality disorder" may be diagnosed if the person seeking their assistance is "humorless or dull." Associated features of their mental disorder also include being "not with it" or "in a fog."[21] Meanwhile, those with histrionic personality disorder "crave novelty, stimulation, and excitement" as they "act out a role, such as the 'victim' or the 'princess'"; those with narcissistic personality disorder "might be more concern[ed] about being seen with the 'right' people than having close friends," and so on.[22] Yet the meetings and memos that generated these diagnoses are, if anything, even more hair-raising.

When the Personality Disorders committee met to redefine passive-aggressive disorder (or PAP, as the psychiatrists began to call it), one committee member, Donald Klein, pushed to make the illness encompass "resistance to demands for *increased activity*."[23] The colleague who opposed him, Steven E. Hyler, did so largely on the basis that Klein evinced similar traits: "I do not interpret Doctor Klein's remarks as stubborn, negativistic, or intentionally inefficient," he declared. "They are much too direct and should probably be classified as oppositional defiant disorder."[24]

Nor was Hyler alone in pathologizing colleagues who disagreed with him. At one particularly tense moment during discussion of the criteria for avoidant personality disorder, Spitzer asked Klein, "Does the reference to 'hypersensitivity to rejection' get too close to Hysteroid Dysphoria for your personal comfort?"[25]

As surprising as it sounds, we are likely in Hyler's debt that indirectly stated doubts about a manager's competence are not considered signs of mental illness. But Hyler's colleagues didn't reject Klein's recommendation completely, they modified it so the "essential feature" of PAP became, in the words of *DSM-III*, "resistance to demands for *adequate performance*; the resistance is expressed indirectly rather than directly."[26] Hyler also made clear that it would be fine to say that a person with the disorder displayed two of these qualities: "indecisivenss [*sic*], lack of assertion, [and] lack of self-confidence."[27] He concluded in parentheses, "perhaps only one of three is sufficient."[28]

Hyler's contribution to the *DSM* fortunately was modest. Five months earlier, he had penned a memo that apparently recommends the inclusion of ailments as vague as "chronic complaint" and "chronic undifferentiated unhappiness" disorders on the basis that a person suffering from the second of these "often present[s] a very sad face," and a person experiencing the first inflicts their "persistent and consistent complaining . . . in a high-pitched whining fashion which is especially noxious to the listener."[29]

It was in describing "chronic complaint disorder," however, that Hyler really found his stride:

To be included in this category are persons who heretofore were known by the synonyms: "kvetch," "scooch," "noodge," and just plain "neurotic."

An episode of acute complaining is usually elicited by the question: "How are you?" The pathognemonic [sic] response is, "Don't ask." The response complaints are of a general nature and include such diverse topics as the weather, the energy crisis, taxes, or the previous evening's track results. . . .

Associated features in this disorder include an outlook on life which is characterized as pessimistic. . . . There also appears to be an ethnic association with this disorder in that it is found predominantly in persons of Eastern-European ancestry. In these cases, the pathognemonic expression becomes, "Oy vay, don't ask."[30]

Hyler's diagnostic zeal might well elicit the same response from readers. But Spitzer was more diplomatic in forwarding the proposal, merely adding in his cover letter, one hopes with irony: "Enclosed are draft versions of two new disorders for possible inclusion in DSM-III . . . It is gratifying to see that the methodology that we have so painstakingly developed for the 'traditional' disorders, applies equally well to disorders yet awaiting discovery."[31] Thereafter, the proposal seems to have generated only bemused or stony silence. If it were all a joke, and Spitzer were somehow in on it, one wishes that Hyler's memo did not so closely resemble the memos he circulated elsewhere about already existing diagnoses.

To its credit, the Advisory Committee on Personality Disorders initially questioned the inclusion of PAP in *DSM-III*, arguing that the latter seemed tied more to situational patterns than personality traits—a symptom of military origins it clearly had outgrown. Their skepticism might have derived from Michael Fielding's insistence that experts could spot the disorder by such clear pathological signs as when a patient "feels misunderstood" while displaying a "negative attitude (chip on shoulder)";[32] or by Ivan Elder's advising them from Tuscaloosa's Veterans Administration Hospital that the "passive-aggressive is *both* too demanding and too dependent," before he listed, as an example of such behavior, "a child 'tak[ing] his (her) marbles home' after the other kids refuse to play 'her (his) way.'"[33]

But Erwin R. Smarr, a psychiatrist serving on the Assembly Liaison Task Force, wasn't happy about removing the illness from the *DSM* and urged Spitzer's committee to reconsider. Drawing on his own experience with veterans, he insisted that the afflicted would "certainly be rightly amazed if psychiatrists could not even recognize that such a pattern existed."[34] In a curious twist, then, patients themselves were said to be crying out for continued recognition of behavior that doesn't, in this case, seem at all passive-aggressive.

Spitzer was at first noncommittal to this objection, conceding, "There has been no outpouring of enthusiasm from this Committee for the inclusion of this category. For some existential reason," he added, "on this matter, I have no personal beliefs other than to exclude the category would certainly cause a lot of bad feeling from this Committee."[35] But he wasn't so indifferent or disinterested as to risk disappointing Smarr; and as Spitzer wrapped up his memo, his tone resumed a pitch he often adopted successfully with many other disorders:

> As you can see from the enclosed letter from Dr. Smarr, a member of the Assembly DSM-III Task Force, he and his group are quite insistent on including this category in *DSM-III*. . . . As Don [Klein] has noted, we have a lot of categories in DSM-III of questionable validity, and I don't think that we should object to trying this category out in the Field Trials. . . . I therefore urge that we include this category in the[m] . . . and see how often it is used. If any of you have strong objections to my gentle twisting of the Advisory Committee's collective arm (arms?), please let me know.[36]

The rationale for extending the life of a disorder first introduced to pathologize stubborn soldiers came down to saying that it wasn't *that* much weaker than a host of other illnesses "of questionable validity." The problem is that Spitzer's team had only agreed about large numbers of *them* because interested parties had greeted their discussion with comparable assurances and appeals.

Worse still, when the APA brought out a revised version of the third edition in 1987 that aimed to tighten the diagnostic criteria of several hazily summarized disorders, the "essential features" of passive-aggressive personality disorder became, if possible, even cloudier than before. In the manual's words:

> When an executive gives a subordinate some material to review for a meeting the next morning, rather than complain that he or she has no time to do the work, the subordinate may misplace or misfile the material and thus attain his or her goal by passively resisting the demand on him.
>
> These people become sulky, irritable, or argumentative when asked to do something they do not want to do. They often protest to others about how unreasonable the demands being made on them are, and resent useful suggestions from others concerning how to be more productive.

And under the heading "impairment," the manual insisted:

> These people are ineffective both socially and occupationally because of their passive-resistant behavior. For example, because of their intentional inefficiency, job promotions are not offered them. A housewife with the disorder may fail to do the laundry or to stock the kitchen with food because of procrastination and dawdling.[37]

The illness, concludes the manual, presents these "associated features": "Often individuals with this disorder are dependent and lack self-confidence. Typically, they are pessimistic about the future but have no realization that their behavior is responsible for their difficulties."[38]

The APA's problems weren't limited to faulty reasoning and ridiculous examples; imprecision was another blemish. In the passage above, "*passive-aggressive*" behavior unaccountably morphs into "passive *resistance*"—a move perhaps due to carelessness or deliberate sleight of hand, but troubling on either score. Passive resistance has a dignified history, dating at least to eighteenth-century Irish dissidents who banded together to reject British Home Rule. The Quakers and eventually Mohandas K. Gandhi adopted similar names for their strategies. Consequently, it is bizarre to see *DSM-IIIR* (in 1987!) declare that such behavior is a disorder typified by such routine traits as "fail[ing] to do the laundry or to stock the kitchen with food because of procrastination and dawdling."

Despite the greatly increased scope of these additions, it is also amazing to report that several psychiatrists actually voiced concern that the disorder was still too "narrowly focused."[39] Others thought it "too situation specific," presumably wanting more locations referenced than the office, the home, and—in *DSM-III*—the club. Their concern was such that the *DSM-IV* task force considered deleting the disorder altogether. But others thought that rash and pressed for a compromise. After Theodore Millon, a consultant on the *DSM-III* task force, recommended renaming the disorder, arguing that "terms such as 'oppositional personality disorder' or 'negativistic personality disorder' capture the flavor of these patients more clearly," his colleagues agreed to "Negativistic (Passive-Aggressive) Personality Disorder" and moved the illness to the handbook's appendix, where it still exists today and looks set to remain after DSM-5 appears.[40]

For some time, as he notes wryly in essays and books, Millon's concern about how to diagnose people with "introverted personalities" went unheeded. (*Whether* to diagnose them was never, for him, in question.) In June 1978, he averred of such people:

I would like to see us make more reference to their characteristic behavioral apathy, their lack of vitality, their deficits in . . . spontaniety [sic], their inability to display enthusiasm or experience pleasure, their minimal introspectiveness and awareness of self, as well as their imperviousness to the subtleties of everyday social life. I think our description and our diagnostic criteria would be strengthened if we included these personality dimensions that clearly signify the disorder.[41]

It may seem peculiar to accuse introverts of "minimal introspectiveness," but, as we'll see, this is not the only matter that is baffling about Millon's work.[42]

When it came to defining the essential features of "Negativistic (Passive-Aggressive) Personality Disorder," his description was quite sweeping:

I would suggest some of the following: frequently irritable and erratically moody; a tendency to report being easily frustrated and angry; discontented self-image, as evidenced in feeling misunderstood and unappreciated by others; characteristically pessimistic, disgruntled and disillusioned with life; interpersonal ambivalence, as evidenced in a struggle between being dependently acquiescent and assertively independent; the use of unpredictable and sulking behaviors to provoke discomfort in others.[43]

"I think each of the above," he concluded, "will enrich the descriptive material we have."

Millon's memo circulated two years before *DSM-III* was published in 1980, but, perhaps because his definition was so scattershot, the *DSM-IV* task force waited thirteen years before it paid much attention to his concerns. In 1991, however, the *DSM-IV Options Book* finally agreed to list the symptoms of Millon's "Negativistic Personality Disorder" alongside those of PAP, to see which should prevail. Millon's lists were so open-ended as to include phrases like, "expresses envy and resentment toward those apparently more fortunate" and "claims to be luckless, ill-starred, and jinxed in life; personal content is more a matter of whining and grumbling than of feeling forlorn and despairing."[44] It was almost as if Hyler had managed to resurrect his proposal for "chronic complaint disorder."

Nevertheless, the published version of *DSM-IV* combined the lists while scaling back some of Millon's more extreme criteria. But the spirit and language of his 1978 memo remained. For instance, the *Options Book* included as potential symptoms "(2) complains of being victimized, misunderstood, and unappreciated by those with whom he or she lives and works," and "(5) communicates a pervasive mix of angry and pessimistic attitudes toward numerous and diverse events (e.g., cynically notes the potentially trouble-some aspects of situations that are not going well)."[45] Only the latter was cut from *DSM-IV*; all of the other options remained, including all but the final clause of "(8) alternates between hostile assertions of personal autonomy and independence, and acting contrite and dependent."[46]

Indeed, *DSM-IV*—though in the appendix—gave arguably the loosest definition of the illness yet, opining:

> These individuals . . . may be sullen, irritable, impatient, argumentative, cynical, skeptical, and contrary. . . . Because of their negativism and ten-dency to externalize blame, the[y] often criticize and voice hostility toward authority figures with minimal provocation. They are also envious and resentful of peers who succeed and who are viewed positively by author-ity figures. These individuals often complain about their personal misfor-tunes. They have a negative view of the future and may make comments such as, "It doesn't pay to be good" and "Good things don't last."[47]

If you are broadly skeptical about those in positions of power, or simply worried about the future and concerned about whether good things can last, you could be diagnosable for the disorder under the terms listed in the appendix. Up until 1994, the disorder had been listed in the main body of the manual, with the all-important diagnostic code, for forty-two years.

Hopefully because of this astonishing description of negativity in the appendix of *DSM-IV*, psychiatrists are still of two minds about what to do with the disorder. Some think it should be dropped entirely from the *DSM*, with Thomas Widiger declaring that it "may already be on the path to extinc-tion."[48] But many more seem to believe it could be rehabilitated if it were slightly redefined. "By renaming and relegating PAPD to the Appendix," assert Scott Wetzler and Leslie C. Morey, "the DSM-IV work group may have sounded its death knell. . . . [But] although it may be difficult to differentiate PAPD from other personality disorders, this is a shortcoming common to all personality disorders. It may not be a ringing endorsement," they concede, "but one can only conclude that PAPD is no less valid than other personality disorders."[49]

One could of course conclude quite differently, using their admission to press that *all* personality disorders be eliminated from the *DSM*. And that would sound reasonable, given the diagnostic criteria we have quoted from published editions of the manual. But few, if any, psychiatrists would agree to that. In a 1992 essay on the disorder's "diagnostic validity," for instance, Mark Fine, James Overholser, and Karen Berkoff acknowledged that the criteria look more promising when viewed from a "dimensional rather than a categorical perspective," but most of their recommendations boiled down to urging their colleagues to recognize their talent for alliteration. Passive-aggressive behavior, they wrote, amounts to a combination of these five elements: "rigidity, resentment, resistance, reactance, and reversed reinforcement."[50]

That was eighteen years ago, and few seemed to heed their advice. The disorder might have languished indefinitely in the Appendix of the *DSM*. But in 2007, a team on the East Coast boldly asserted "The Validity of DSM-IV Passive-Aggressive (Negativistic) Personality Disorder," while lamenting incredulously that "the diagnosis has never gained international acceptance."[51] Their article amounts to a concerted push to revive it in altered (negativistic) form and to let it shine once more among all the other personality, mood, and anxiety disorders in the *DSM*.

To do that, the authors focus on the disorder's "long history" without acknowledging its surprising twists and turns, including that it recently acquired a new name and has been expanded beyond all recognition. But their main contribution is to offer "empirical data" on a disorder that hitherto was surprisingly lacking in such data.[52]

At first blush, their data look impressive. The authors draw from a sample of 1,200 psychiatric outpatients at Rhode Island Hospital, and state that, of these patients, thirty-five participants (3.02 percent) "met criteria" for Passive-Aggressive (Negativistic) Personality Disorder (NEGPD). Incidentally, most of the patients were white; over half of them were women; and almost half of the patients were married.

Pages of data follow, including tables itemizing "convergent and divergent validity coefficients for Negativistic Personality Disorder criteria" and "Axis II Comorbidity in Patients with and without Negativistic Personality Disorder." But when listing the criteria in question, the illusion of scientific precision unfortunately bursts. The criteria, as one should expect from *DSM-IV*, include "[feels] misunderstood and unappreciated"; "[experiences] envy and resentment"; "[regrets] personal misfortune," and so on. To that end, when trying to draw bold pointers from their data, the authors are reduced to making absurd statements like the following: "The data showed that 'complaints of being misunderstood and unappreciated' and 'sullen and argumentative' were the most correlated to the NEGPD criteria set. Additionally, the item 'voices exaggerated . . . complaints of personal misfortune' was the most diagnostically efficient."[53] But, really, wouldn't it have to be? This must be, after all, one of the most rampant grumbles going.

Psychiatrists may wince over these passages, insisting that passive-aggressive disorder since *DSM-IV* has been shorn of cachet, so there's no point in dredging up its unillustrious career. Or they may persist, as the authors above do, in saying that skepticism and petulance are really symptoms of a bona fide illness. But as a close study of almost any disorder in the *DSM* would likely yield the same cringing results, in recording what happened to passive-aggressive disorder—just one of over 350 disorders sharing quite similar histories—I am also bringing to light a significant and largely unexamined chapter of American psychiatry.

The letters and memos reprinted here point to the APA's widespread difficulty in distinguishing between normal and pathological behavior. This is not a trivial problem when the organization's manual is invoked daily around the world by courts, prisons, schools, and mental health professionals of every stripe. Such difficulties and their knock-on effects also encourage us to ask how much faith we can or should place in the current *DSM* task force, which is now meeting to assemble the next edition of psychiatry's bible, *DSM-5*. According to early reports from the APA, *DSM-5* is likely to add "temper dysregulation," "mixed anxiety," "hypersexual disorder," "psychosis risk syndrome," and "internet addiction disorder" to the diagnostic manual, with the latter appearing in its appendix as a condition awaiting further research. As of this writing (April 2010), *DSM-5* is also likely to redefine the personality disorders by trait domains and trait facets, with those of PAPD marked by "oppositionality, hostility, and guilt/shame."[54] At that rate, perhaps we shouldn't be surprised if "dissent" itself becomes one of the disorder's "trait domains" and belief that "Good things don't last" returns as one of its distinguishing symptoms.

NOTES

1. All unpublished correspondence cited in this chapter appears courtesy of the American Psychiatric Association in Arlington, Virginia, for which I thank Gary McMillan. A slightly different version appeared in the journal *Theory and Psychology.* Georges Canguilhem, *The Normal and the Pathological,* trans. Carolyn R. Fawcett with Robert S. Cohen, intro. Michel Foucault (New York: Zone Books, 1991), esp. 275–87. See also Foucault, *Psychiatric Power: Lectures at the Collège de France, 1973-1974,* ed. Jacques Lagrange, trans. Graham Burchell (New York: Palgrave Macmillan, 2006), esp. 265–95.

2. Peter D. Kramer, *Listening to Prozac: The Landmark Book about Antidepressants and the Remaking of the Self,* rev. ed. (New York: Penguin, 1997), 15.

3. I elaborate fully on the practical and financial details of this campaign in *Shyness: How Normal Behavior Became a Sickness* (New Haven: Yale University Press, 2007), chap. 4. See also Samuel M. Turner, Deborah C. Beidel, and Ruth M. Townsley, "Social Phobia: Relationship to Shyness," *Behaviour Research and Therapy* 28, no. 6 (1990): esp. 497.

4. David C. Rettew, "Avoidant Personality Disorder, Generalized Social Phobia, and Shyness: Putting the Personality Back into the Personality Disorders," *Harvard Review of Psychiatry* 8, no. 6 (December 2000): 285.

5. Ronald C. Kessler, Patricia Berglund, Olga Demler, Robert Jin, Kathleen R. Merikangas, and Ellen E. Walters, "Lifetime Prevalence and Age-of-Onset Distributions of *DSM-IV* Disorders in the National Comorbidity Survey Replication," *Archives of General Psychiatry* 62, no. 6 (June 2005): 593.

6. David Healy and Graham Aldred, "Antidepressant Drug Use and the Risk of Suicide," *International Review of Psychiatry* 17, no. 3 (June 2005): 168.

7. Marcela Gaviria, producer of *The Medicated Child* (2008) for PBS's *Frontline* TV series, cites this percentage in an interview about her documentary. See Ada Calhoun, "Toddlers Medicated for Bipolar Disorder in Record Numbers," *AOL News*, January 8, 2008, http://news.aol.com/newsbloggers/2008/01/08/record-number-of-toddlers-medicated-for-bipolar-disorder/.

8. See for instance Herb Kutchins and Stuart A. Kirk, *Making Us Crazy: DSM: The Psychiatric Bible and the Creation of Mental Disorders* (New York: Free Press, 1997).

9. Dr. William C. Menninger, "Bulletin TB M.D. 203, dated October 19, 1945," cited in Kenneth L. Malinow, "Passive-Aggressive Personality," in *Personality Disorders: Diagnosis and Management, Second Edition,* ed. John R. Lion (Baltimore: Williams and Wilkins, 1981), 123.

10. Cecil Adams, "What Is 'Passive-Aggressive?'" *The Straight Dope*, May 30, 2003, http://www.straightdope.com/columns/030530.html.

11. James R. Hodge, Lt. (MC) USNR, "The Passive-Dependent versus the Passive-Aggressive Personality," *Unites States Armed Forces Medical Journal* 6, no. 1 (1955): 87.

12. Ibid., 85.

13. American Psychiatric Association, Committee on Nomenclature and Statistics, *Mental Disorders; Diagnostic and Statistical Manual (DSM-I)* (Washington, DC: American Psychiatric Association, 1952), 37 (000–x52).

14. See for instance Thomas F. McGee and Thaddeus Kostrubala, "The Neurotic Equilibrium in Married Couples Applying for Group Psychotherapy," *Journal of Marriage and the Family* 26, no. 1 (February 1964): 77–82. About one man, the authors write, "Psychological testing . . . suggested that he would like to relate to women in a passive-dependent manner but saw them as aggressive, destructive, and controlling. This did not deter him from over attempts to establish a passive-dependent relationship with women. The diagnosis was that he was a passive-aggressive personality, passive-dependent type" (81).

15. Stefan A. Pasternak, "The Explosive, Antisocial, and Passive-Aggressive Personalities," *Personality Disorders: Diagnosis and Management,* ed. John R. Lion (Baltimore: Williams and Wilkins, 1974), 63. Pasternak's essay does not appear in the second edition of this collection, cited in note 9.

16. *DSM-I*, 36 (000–x51) and 38 (000–x60).

17. American Psychiatric Association, Committee on Nomenclature and Statistics, *Diagnostic and Statistical Manual of Mental Disorders,* 2nd ed. (*DSM-II*) (Washington, DC: American Psychiatric Association, 1968), 41–42 (301).

18. Ibid., 44 (301.81).

19. Robert L. Spitzer, Michael Sheehy, and Jean Endicott, "*DSM-III*: Guiding Principles," in *Psychiatric Diagnosis,* ed. Vivian M. Rakoff, Harvey C. Stancer, and Henry B. Kedward (New York: Brunner/Mazel, 1977), 1.

20. American Psychiatric Association, Committee on Nomenclature and Statistics, *Diagnostic and Statistical Manual of Mental Disorders,* 3rd ed. (*DSM-III*) (Washington, DC: American Psychiatric Association, 1980), 329 (301.84).

21. Ibid., 310 (301.20).

22. Ibid., 313 (301.50) and 316 (301.81).

23. Donald F. Klein, "Personality Disorders—Passive-Aggressive Personality," as quoted by Steven E. Hyler, "Passive-Aggressive Personality Disorder Critique by Dr. D. Klein," October 31, 1977.

24. Hyler to Spitzer, October 31, 1977.

25. Spitzer to Klein, February 27, 1978.

26. *DSM-III* 328 (301.84).

27. Hyler to Spitzer, October 31, 1977.

28. Ibid.

29. Hyler to Spitzer, May 10, 1977.

30. Ibid.

31. Robert Spitzer to the DSM-III task force, May 10, 1977.

32. Michael F. Fielding, memo on Passive-Aggressive Personality Disorder, May 11, 1978.

33. Ivan Elder to Robert Spitzer, March 14, 1978; emphasis in original.

34. Erwin R. Smarr to Spitzer and Hector Jason, chair of the Assembly Liaison Task Force on DSM-III, November 4, 1977.

35. Spitzer to the Advisory Committee on Personality Disorders, November 9, 1977.

36. Ibid.

37. American Psychiatric Association, Committee on Nomenclature and Statistics, *Diagnostic and Statistical Manual of Mental Disorders,* 3rd ed. rev. (*DSM-IIIR*) (Washington, DC: American Psychiatric Association, 1987), 356–57 (301.84).

38. Ibid., 357.

39. Theodore (Ted) Millon to the Advisory Committee on Personality Disorders, June 28, 1978.

40. Ibid.

41. Ibid.

42. See for instance his *Disorders of Personality: DSM-III, Axis II* (New York: Wiley, 1981), 252, 246. Here, he argues that there's likely a "biological" reason passive-aggressives exude "a capricious impulsiveness, an irritable moodiness, a grumbling, discontented, sulky, unaccommodating, and fault-finding pessimism that characterizes their behaviors. . . . Even in the best of circumstances," he despairs, "they always seem to seek the 'dark lining in the silver cloud.'"

43. Ibid.

44. American Psychiatric Association, Task Force on DSM-IV, *DSM-IV Options Book: Work in Progress* (Washington, DC: American Psychiatric Association, 1991), R:17

45. Ibid. Compare these with the research criteria published for "Passive-Aggressive Personality Disorder (Negativistic Personality Disorder)," in the appendix of *DSM-IV,* 735. The phrasing is almost identical.

46. Ibid.

47. *DSM-IV*, 733–34.

48. Thomas A. Widiger, "Personality Disorder and Axis I Psychopathology: The Problematic Boundary of Axis I and Axis II," *Journal of Personality Disorders* 17, no. 2 (2003): 98.

49. Scott Wetzler and Leslie C. Morey, "Passive-Aggressive Personality Disorder: The Demise of a Syndrome," *Psychiatry* 62, no. 1 (1999): 57.

50. Mark A. Fine, James C. Overholser, and Karen Berkoff, "Diagnostic Validity of the Passive-Aggressive Personality Disorder: Suggestions for Reform," *American Journal of Psychotherapy* 46, no. 3 (1992): 470, 478.

51. Ora H. Rotenstein, Wilson McDermut, Andrea Bergman, Diane Young, Mark Zimmerman, and Iwona Chelminski, "The Validity of DSM-IV Passive-Aggressive (Negativistic) Personality Disorder," *Journal of Personality Disorders* 21, no. 1 (2007): 30.

52. Ibid., 30.

53. Ibid., 38.

54. I discuss this problem more extensively in "Bitterness, Compulsive Shopping, and Internet Addiction: The Diagnostic Madness of *DSM-V*," *Slate*, July 24, 2009, http://www.slate.com/id/2223479/.

Obsession

Against Mental Health

——————————————————————— LENNARD J. DAVIS ———

Obsessive-compulsive disorder (OCD) was a rare and strange disease before the 1970s. Estimates of its prevalence in the general population at that time were from 0.05 percent to 0.005 percent.[1] If you were a mental health practitioner, you would expect to see, by the former percentage, one person out of two thousand who had the disorder, or by the latter, one person in every twenty thousand. In 1973, a researcher could write that OCD was "unquestionably, one of the rarest forms of mental disorders."[2] Consequently, if you were a person with severe symptoms of OCD in the mid-1970s, you would probably assume that you were alone, odd, and certainly crazy. You might even have been treated as someone who straddled the borderline between neurosis and psychosis.

In the intervening years, OCD has gone from a rare and intractable illness, perhaps requiring brain surgery, to a quite common, routinely diagnosed, and treatable disorder. The ambient, cultural world has become peopled with loveable images of OCD from Tony Shaloub on the TV series *Monk* to Jack Nicholson in the film *As Good as It Gets*. Most estimates now say that 2 to 3 percent of the population will have OCD during their lifetimes; that is two or three out of every hundred. Recent attempts to describe an OCD spectrum increase the incidence to one in ten.[3]

How did we go from one out of twenty thousand to three out of a hundred to one in ten in less than thirty years? An extremely rare disease has now become rampant. Indeed, the World Health Organization's 2001 mental health report noted that "Four other mental disorders figure in the top 10 causes of disability in the world, namely alcohol abuse, bipolar disorder, schizophrenia and obsessive compulsive disorder."[4] So now OCD is one of the top four mental disorders in the world. Consequently, it has become one of the most researched disorders.[5]

Any simple psychiatric definition of OCD or explanation for the uptick in the prevalence of the disorder is bound to be reductionist. It's not simply that scientists are by definition simpleminded, but that medicine tends to want to find *the* single cause for an illness. However, with OCD the explanation can only be complex. This isn't to say that contemporary explanations of OCD aren't complex and even interdisciplinary, but because they inevitably leave out the crucial social, historical, and cultural elements—the biocultural part of the disease—and fail to examine their own methods, biases, and premises, these explanations will necessarily be incomplete.

Researchers and the general public broadly assume that to be pro-health means that a practitioner listens to, tests, and observes a patient, thumbs mentally through a range of diagnoses, and picks the appropriate disease. But this pro-health stance might actually be an anti-health one because diagnoses for mental disorders themselves might be something less than clear and obvious. It is possible, I argue here, that to diagnose a person with a psychiatric disorder using available categories might be against health.

There is a general tendency to assume that professionals and practitioners, particularly if their expertise is in the sciences, have arrived at the definitive concept or idea of a phenomenon.[6] Science, unlike the humanities, discards previous knowledge in favor of the most current (and presumably correct) explanation. Yet histories of science and medicine are only optional knowledges for working scientists. Experts in OCD may believe they have little need of the kind of genealogy I am suggesting. The complex knowledge offered in this book and by those who are investigating how some practices in medicine can be against health, however, may signal a way out of this diagnostic straitjacket. To not very lyrically paraphrase Yeats, how can you know the disease from the history of the disease or the person with OCD from the disorder?

OCD: Disease or Disease Entity?

The first major issue to consider in any in-depth, biocultural study of OCD is whether the constellation of behaviors and thought patterns that we are calling OCD is a coherent and freestanding one. In other words, are we looking at a disease or a disease entity? When the *Diagnostic and Statistical Manual of Mental Disorders* (*DSM*) was first established in 1952, it modified the historical notion of OCD by separating phobias from obsessions and establishing the obsessive-compulsive personality as distinct from the disorder itself.[7] In 1968, the *DSM-II* codified that distinction between personality and disorder. Each subsequent edition has further modified the criteria for the disease, defining OCD as something separate from schizophrenia or depression and increasing the time required for the diagnosis from three weeks to six weeks. The next edition may include the idea of an OCD spectrum. Each of these changes makes an alteration to the disease entity, to the number of people who have the illness, and by extension to the social impact of the disorder.

Have we reached the end of the line now? Are we looking at the cumulative corrections of a process of trial and error? Or is the entity we now call OCD just as much of a disease made by committee as it has been in the past? Michael Stone notes that "No matter how tightly and rigorously we define OCD in contemporary psychiatry, there is still conceptual overlap with various 'diagnostic near-neighbors.'" He notes that our definition can take on "the coloration of delusion . . . and there is no fine line demarcating *compulsion* from *impulsion* such as to rid these concepts satisfactorily of an overlap." Furthermore, "the common 'fellow-travelers' of OCD (phobia, panic, depression) and the fairly wide range of severity among bona fide cases of OCD will ensure a level of semantic confusion well beyond our day."[8] Another way of saying this is that OCD may not be a discrete, separate entity at all. One researcher notes that 77 percent of his OCD patients have a lifetime history of another Axis I disorder, while 57 percent who came to a clinic had at least one other Axis I *DSM-III-R* diagnosis.[9] Given the current pitch of research on functional brain activity, neurochemical transactions, and genetic locations, we have to ask if the category OCD is itself something discrete enough to plug into a scientific equation. For example, if there are likely to be two disorders in the brains of OCD patients as was just noted, how can any neurological test find the single place or problem causing OCD? If there are gradients and continua in the disease, how can there be a specific area in the brain that causes the specific response we are calling OCD? Furthermore, the problem of defining OCD is more difficult in children, as much of what children do is obsessive. As Paul Adams writes, "obsession is everywhere, in all of us. Among children, it characterizes a life style, or a transient and recoverable state, or an unrelenting neurosis, or a severe psychotic illness, or a collective 'game.' Obsessive behavior appears all along a broad and diverse spectrum of childhood activities."[10] It is true that most researchers in OCD acknowledge that they are always refining and fine-tuning the diagnosis. *DSM-V* may remove the concept of obsessive personality disorder entirely and introduce the notion of an "obsessive-compulsive continuum." But is what they are left with a freestanding entity?

If, as it is argued by many current researchers, the disease is a structural and chemical disorder, then by definition it can't be a disease that is the result of societal or familial or even individual pressures. That is to say, if you have a broken leg, it doesn't matter to the diagnosis if you are rich or poor, have had a happy or sad childhood, and so on; likewise, if you have a broken brain, other factors matter much less as well. To buttress this idea of the inherent and biologically universal nature of OCD, many clinical and popular books on the disorder claim that the illness has been around since time immemorial. In such books there are cursory references to tenth-century Persians, Paracelsus, medieval and Renaissance physicians, Lady Macbeth, Dr. Johnson, Catholic Church concerns with religious scrupulosity, and a smattering of other examples. Based on this slim evidence, the claim remains that OCD has always been around, and further, that it is found in all cultures. Each book that is published—whether clinical or self-help—repeats these snippets of proof in an introductory paragraph or two. Yet the actual historical evidence for the existence of OCD is scant and would not stand up to scrutiny in a freshman history class. We might want to consider this belief in the historical continuity of OCD as part of an origination myth for those who now research the disorder.

In addition to the "it's always been around" myth is the putative global nature of OCD. That claim is equally grand although the evidence again is scant, based mainly on a cross-national epidemiological study of Canada, Puerto Rico, Germany, Taiwan, Korea, and New Zealand which showed OCD to be present in all those countries except Taiwan.[11] Though widely cited, this study is actually a review article that looks at varying data over a rather long period of time in a mere six countries and the United States. This hardly represents a survey of the world. A few further epidemiological studies are used to make the global claim. A typical example of how this claim works can be found in a chapter of an influential book on OCD. There, the author states that "The basic types and frequencies of obsessive-compulsive symptoms are consistent across cultures and time."[12] Two footnotes with references are provided. One is a study of the prevalence of OCD in Japan and the other on "preliminary psychiatric observations" in Egypt. These two articles are the sole basis for the rather sweeping claim that OCD symptoms are consistent across all cultures and times!

Epidemiological analyses have been complicated by the fact that "an optimal threshold or diagnostic criterion that reliably distinguishes the clinical from the subthreshold syndrome of OCD has yet to be identified."[13] What this means is that it's hard to identify when the kind of obsessive behaviors that might be part of our culture cross over into a disease entity. A high percentage of people in the normal population have obsessions and compulsions that are indistinguishable in content from those who are defined as clinical, with frequency and intensity being the distinguishing factors.[14] A standard tool used to determine if someone has OCD is the Yale-Brown Obsessive Compulsive Scale (Y-BOCS). But with this test, as with any other, a numerical threshold has to be identified above which you have the disease and below which you don't. In some cases, the cut-off is a score of sixteen, but others argue for a cut-off of twenty.[15]

The questionnaire used by the cross-national study of OCD, for example, seems far from objective. The questions are leading, repetitive, and unsubtle.[16] Moreover, there are methodological questions. The study has been critiqued for using non-professional, untrained interviewers in some countries. Without highly trained staff, any series of questions like these can be shaped by the tone, voice, and manner of the interviewer, who would clearly be happy to get positive answers. Given all this, it's not surprising that this study elicited a large number of positives for people identified as having OCD. Furthermore, how well were the translations of the Y-BOCS checklist tested to assure that they would be standardized from language to language? Finally, which groups of people were tested? Did they include homeless people, prisoners, the poor? If not, the study might reflect the interests of middle-class people and those more likely to be involved in such a study in the first place.

If this seminal study, so widely cited, is full of holes, how can it be used to justify the claim of the global universality of OCD? As opposed to this universal existence of OCD, it is possible to make a specific argument about the disorder's shifting and changing symptoms and photograph these symptoms for a moment in the framing of the concept itself. If we buy this explanation, it becomes quite difficult to argue, in the current mode of research and reasoning, that a specific region of the brain or a specific arrangement of neurotransmitters is ultimately responsible for the occurrence of OCD. You can of course argue that a specific area of the brain may be involved in worrying or planning or checking, but to assume that the brain has a specific location or set of locations for something that itself is not fixed or universal is a deeply problematic assumption. In other words, if there isn't a locked box that contains OCD and only OCD, then any attempt to find the exact site of something like OCD will be a flawed endeavor. It would be like trying to find the place in the brain or the neurochemistry behind the desire to drink a Starbucks latte rather than a Dunkin' Donuts regular.[17]

In arguing for a more complex explanation and understanding of disease entities, I am not saying that attempts to locate the part of the brain in which OCD lives or the chemicals through which it may function are futile endeavors. Indeed, we need to understand the mechanisms of the brain in much better detail, and that prospect is an exciting and complex one. But I am saying that these investigations are only part of the story, and that the larger story is not an irrelevant part of the formation of the concept of the disorder itself. When I've presented talks to practitioners and researchers, I see that many are receptive to the historical information I provide. But they walk away not really believing that knowing the biocultural aura of facts and effects that surround a disease entity has much, if any, value in their study of the specific neurological mechanisms of OCD. If you are trying to find a defective spark plug, knowing the history of the development of the car seems irrelevant at worst and at best, merely entertaining. But if you are trying to figure out how and why a particular car got to Philadelphia, simply understanding how the spark plug works won't help you. You will need to know the life story of the driver and her current wishes and desires. What I'm saying is that trying to understand OCD is more like trying to figure out how a car got to Philadelphia and the approach being taken by researchers is more like trying to figure out how a spark plug functions.

If your model of OCD is that it is based on an imbalance of neurotransmitters or a malfunction of the basal ganglia, if yours is a broken-brain model, then you have a static model of the disorder. In your static scenario, you will see the human mechanism as consistently the same—steady throughout all history—and presume that the factors that lead to OCD are, by definition, distinctly organic and ahistorical. Environmental factors will be of some interest, but they will generally be seen as universal ones like those that lead to a strep infection or the mechanisms of stress.

If the past is any predictor, the universal model is inadequate for a number of reasons. A central one is that if you locate a brain region, a neurotransmitter, or a genetic region—or all three—you will still only be able to attribute that cause to a fraction of the total people with OCD. You will then be able to say something like 30 percent of people with OCD have a pattern of Single Nucleotide Polymorphisms (SNPs) in a particular gene. But how can you then explain the 70 percent that do not?[18] If the universal, ahistorical notion of a broken brain that needs repair were accurate, an account like this should describe *all* sufferers, not a fraction of them.

In addition, if you adhere to this universal and static model, you will have difficulty in explaining why OCD was a relatively rare disease before the 1970s and is a relatively common one now. You will have to say that it was simply under-diagnosed in the past. But that explanation will be inadequate because of the ridiculously dramatic upsurge in numbers—anywhere from a forty-fold to a six-hundred-fold increase.[19] Advocates of the universal model argue that OCD is by nature easy to conceal. Yet the *DSM* definition emphasizes that the rituals and behaviors characteristic of the disease do not alone define the disease. What really defines OCD as a disorder is anguish and "marked distress," the ego-dystonic nature of the beast. And so it is a diagnostic and conceptual contradiction to say that something that can be easily concealed is to be known diagnostically by a very palpable anguish and despair, as this pain is by definition not likely to be repressed. It is also noted that OCD causes great concern and anguish to family members.[20] This also indicates that the easy concealment argument isn't so easy at all. I'm not denying that OCD can be kept secret, but that alone cannot explain why suddenly so many more people have OCD.

Another explanation used by many researchers to explain the uptick in diagnoses is that media exposure has allowed people to come forward. When they see OCD portrayed or discussed on television, people may identify their own behaviors and report to physicians that the puzzling things they have been doing have a diagnostic name. There is a lot of truth to the media-exposure theory, but again, it can't fully explain the 40–600 percent upturn in OCD cases. And to the extent that it is true, it is true for many other cognitive and affective disorders as well. How much of the uptick phenomenon is driven by the very researchers and practitioners who then marvel at the increased numbers? It is more likely that family members now have available to them a medicalized narrative about the strange or annoying behavior of their family member. Medicalized narratives are culturally laden and not to be lightly confused with neurological or biochemical explanations of brain functions.

There is a book to be written following the phenomenon of the development of new lifestyle diseases. Indeed, a general trend toward the medicalization of virtually every emotional and cognitive state is upon us.[21] Within the past fifteen years we've seen attention deficit disorder, depression, bipolar disorder, insomnia, restless-leg syndrome, sexual dysfunction, social anxiety disorder, and autism, among others, go from being either unknown or relatively uncommon occurrences to major illnesses. It isn't the role of this chapter to document that larger change, but I do want to suggest that the media explanation isn't without its own complexities.[22] And media exposure actually provides a viewpoint to the way that medical practice and corporate communication media are deeply connected, so much so that they feed into an against-health scenario.

The standard aspect of all these stories is that researchers find a correlation between a certain behavioral/affective structure and a drug or treatment. Studies are done in which a formerly untreatable, or in some cases unknown, disease entity responds to the drug or treatment in question. Initially, these studies are wildly optimistic, although few if any are randomized, double-blind studies. Many are conducted by enthusiastic researchers who are excited about finding a correlation and helping their patients. And let us not forget that careers can be made, funding received, pharmaceuticals developed, and tenure secured around such successes. The initial surge of studies on treatment for OCD with Anafranil cited a 70 percent improvement rate. That 70 percent rate was also cited in initial studies on SSRI treatment for depression. Yet there is an inevitable falloff from these initial, wildly optimistic accounts. In the course of this enthusiasm, researchers publish their work in journals and practitioners read the work and give it a try on their patients. TV, print media, and Websites tout the cure, inform about the new diagnosis, and people—often family members and friends of the newly afflicted— suggest visits to doctors' offices for diagnosis and treatment. A sociology of disease recognition needs to be developed to account for this phenomenon.

As part of this process, researchers will mention that previous regimens were ineffective. The current literature on OCD has a standard narrative that includes the difficulty of treating the disorder, the high failure rate in the past, the poor prognosis, and then the good news of how well the current paradigm is working—not perfect, to be sure, but much more effective. Were things so bad in the past? The reality of obsession in the past could in fact be substantially different. One researcher in the supposedly benighted 1950s says that 39 percent of the people with OCD showed a good prognosis, while 30 percent did not worsen. That would be a total of 69 percent who either improved or stayed the same. Another researcher in 1973, citing this work, suggested "that the natural outcome of untreated cases of obsession in childhood is good."[23] We might want to look with suspicion on how the current moment characterizes the past.

The print media is a very influential means of reaching the lay public, particularly those whom public relations experts call "the influencers," the people who are most likely to have an effect on those around them. Eric Hollander notes that 28 percent of OCD patients came for help as the result of reading, 16 percent by hearing about it on TV or radio.[24] Self-help books on OCD, written by experts or celebrities, bring home the message surrounding the disease entity. These books are always written around a new cure, which the expert touts as the breakthrough that will change things forever.

Most popular books and much of the clinical literature on OCD begin by describing the upsurge in numbers of people with OCD. For example, Judith L. Rapoport, whose best-selling 1989 book *The Boy Who Couldn't Stop Washing* brought OCD to national prominence, observes:

> The textbooks had told us the disease was very rare. Later we came to see how common the problem really was . . . [our] surveys showed that Obsessive-Compulsive Disorder is not at all rare—it is indeed common. Then it quickly became clear that there were treatments that worked. Suddenly, OCD became the psychiatric disease of the 1980s. We began to see many, many patients.[25]

This explosion of OCD is also noted by Lee Baer, who in 1991 wrote:

> When we established the OCD Clinic at Massachusetts General in 1983 . . . I had seen fewer than fifty OCD patients. . . . since then we have seen almost a thousand, and eight new patients now come to our clinic each week. Our colleagues tell us that similar growth has occurred at other OCD clinics around the country.[26]

The magical narrative in which there are no active agents, merely effects, is repeated here and throughout the tale of OCD. Another book written around ten years later observes that OCD, "previously considered a very rare mental disorder, now appears to be a hidden epidemic. Recent research indicates that over 6.5 million people suffer from OCD, making it one of the most common mental disorders . . . [and it] impacts about one adult in 40."[27] The term "hidden epidemic" was echoed in the pages of *The New England Journal of Medicine* when Michael A. Jenike wrote his editorial, "Obsessive-Compulsive and Related Disorders: A Hidden Epidemic."[28] Hollander repeats the term in his article "Obsessive-Compulsive Disorder: The Hidden Epidemic" in *The Journal of Clinical Psychiatry*.[29] He says, "We have overcome the myth that OCD is a rare, untreatable, and psychologically driven disorder."[30] And the title of one self-help book is *Tormenting Thoughts and Secret Rituals: The Hidden Epidemic of Obsessive-Compulsive Disorder.* What exactly is a "hidden epidemic"? It turns out that "hidden epidemic" is virtually a code phrase used to launch public relations campaigns for new disorders. A casual Google search of the term yields the hidden epidemics of autism, depression, bipolar disorder, sexually transmitted diseases, celiac disease, asthma, chronic fatigue syndrome, hepatitis C, drug addiction, sexual violence, obesity, dissociation disorder, birth defects, heart disease, and, of course, concussions in rugby as well as foot-and-mouth disease.

If we don't accept the magical forty-to-six-hundred-fold increase in OCD as an agent-less process, how can we explain it? One could argue that the old 0.05 percent number includes under-reporting, but it also might include the most intractable and severe cases of OCD. The culture had not yet been fully prepared to medicalize a range of behaviors under the terms of OCD. Let us presume that the researchers were in some sense responsible for the formulating and publicizing of the disorder, and that the swelling numbers followed a pattern typical for the emergence of new disease entities. The first phase would be the "discovery" of and publication on the disease along with the new cures, which are wildly effective. Then there is an inevitable seepage from people with the most severe cases to less severe ones. We have seen this "me-too" process come about in the examples of depression and ADD. In those cases, only a small percentage of the population saw themselves as fitting the diagnosis, but later more and more people considered themselves to fit under the diagnostic rubric.[31] As practitioners become part of the process, people self-identify—with or without the encouragement of friends and family—and practitioners prescribe the medications that the patients themselves know of through the media and often request from their doctors.

Could there be a relationship between the initial rarity of OCD and its lack of treatability and the proliferation of the disease and its more successful cure rate? An argument could be made that the people who are more treatable are the newer, less serious cases. One thing that remains a problem for OCD, even with successful treatments, is the rather low rate of cure and the reality that the disorder is chronic. The aim of most practitioners is to reduce the severity and the frequency of symptoms, not to eliminate the disorder, which in many cases seems incurable.

What I've tried to show is that our definitions of mental health can be driven by complex biocultural factors. From understanding the history of a disease entity to conceptualizing and treating various behaviors and conditions, health is something that belongs to the promoters of an explanation as well as those who oppose that explanation. To be against an explanation or a set of explanations doesn't mean that one is against health. Likewise, to be for a set of procedures and diagnoses can be a way of being against health as well. In the end, simplistic and reductionist explanations of complex medical phenomena will always be against health.

1. Michael A. Jenike, Lee Baer, and William Minichiello, eds., *Obsessive-Compulsive Disorders: Practical Management* (St. Louis: Mosby, 1998), 4. See also Paul L. Adams, *Obsessive Children: A Sociopsychiatric Study* (New York: Brunner/Mazel, 1973), 17.

2. Adams, *Obsessive Children*, 17.

3. Eric Hollander, "Obsessive-Compulsive Disorder: The Hidden Epidemic," *Journal of Clinical Psychiatry* 58, no. 12 (1997): 4.

4. *Mental Health: A Call for Action by World Health Ministers* (Geneva: World Health Organization, 2001), 16.

5. Jenike, Baer, and Minichiello, *Obsessive-Compulsive Disorders*, xvi.

6. See Barbara Herrnstein Smith, *Scandalous Knowledge: Science, Truth and the Human* (Durham: Duke University Press, 2006); and Donna Jean Haraway, *ModestWitness@Second Millennium.FemaleManMeetsOncoMouse* (New York: Routledge, 1997).

7. For a much more in-depth consideration of this topic, see my *Obsession: A History* (Chicago: University of Chicago Press, 2008).

8. Michael Stone, introduction to *Essential Papers on Obsessive-Compulsive Disorder*, ed. Dan J. Stein and Michael H. Stone (New York: NYU Press, 1997), 23–24.

9. Steven A. Rasmussen and Jane L. Eisen, "The Epidemiology and Clinical Features of Obsessive-Compulsive Disorder," in Jenike, Baer, and Minichiello, *Obsessive-Compulsive Disorders*, 31.

10. Adams, *Obsessive Children*, 9–10.

11. Myrna M. Weissman, Roger C. Bland et al., "The Cross National Epidemiology of Obsessive Compulsive Disorder," *Journal of Clinical Psychiatry* 55, Supplement (March 1994): 5–10.

12. Rasmussen and Eisen, in Jenike, Baer, and Minichiello, *Obsessive-Compulsive Disorders*, 25.

13. Ibid., 16.

14. S. Rachman and P. DeSilva, "Abnormal and Normal Obsessions," *Behavior Research Therapy* 16, no. 4 (1978): 233–48.

15. See John H. Greist, James W. Jefferson, Kenneth A. Kobak, David J. Katzelnick, and Ronald C. Serlin, "Efficacy and Tolerability of Serotonin Transport Inhibitors in Obsessive-Compulsive Disorder: A Meta-Analysis," *Archives of General Psychiatry* 52, no. 1 (January 1995): 53–60.

16. For a more detailed critique, see my *Obsession: A History*.

17. Not that this hasn't been tried. See Brian Knutson, Scott Rick, G. Elliott Wimmer, Drazen Prelec, and George Loewenstein, "Neural Predictors of Purchases," *Neuron* 53, no. 1 (January 4, 2007): 147–56, as well as Dharol Tankersley, C. Jill Stowe, and Scott A. Huettel, "Altruism Is Associated with an Increased Neural Response to Agency," *Nature Neuroscience* 10, no. 2 (February 2007): 150–51.

18. While there is much enthusiasm for trying to establish a genetic basis for OCD and other mental disorders, that very process needs greater scrutiny. The possibilities for this research are enhanced by computer technologies that allow great computing power to scan massive numbers of SNPs. However, the ease with which this can be done permits a kind of sloppy science that coordinates any set of SNPs with any set of disorders.

19. Dana J. H. Neihaus and Dan J. Stein, "Obsessive-Compulsive Disorder: Diagnosis and Assessment," in *Obsessive-Compulsive Disorders: Diagnosis, Etiology, Treatment*, ed. Eric Hollander and Dan J. Stein (New York: Marcel Dekker, 1997), 2.

20. See, for example, Stanley Rachman, Ray Hodgson, and Isaac M. Marks, "The Treatment of Obsessive-Compulsive Neurosis," cited in Stein and Stone, *Essential Papers*, 203.

21. See H. Gilbert Welch, Lisa Schwartz, and Steven Woloshin, "What's Making Us Sick Is an Epidemic of Diagnoses," *New York Times*, January 2, 2007, http://www.nytimes.com/2007/01/02/health/02essa.html.

22. For accounts of this, see David Healy, *Let Them Eat Prozac: The Unhealthy Relationship Between the Pharmaceutical Industry and Depression* (New York: NYU Press, 2004), as well as his *The Creation of Psychopharmacology* (Cambridge, MA: Harvard University Press, 2002). See too Meika Loe, *The Rise of Viagra: How the Little Blue Pill Changed Sex in America* (New York: NYU Press, 2004).

23. Adams, *Obsessive Children*, 209.

24. Hollander, "Obsessive-Compulsive Disorder," 4.

25. Judith L. Rapoport, *The Body Who Couldn't Stop Washing: The Experience and Treatment of Obsessive-Compulsive Disorder* (New York: Signet, 1991), 13, 8.

26. Lee Baer, *Getting Control: Overcoming Your Obsessions and Compulsions* (Boston: Little, Brown, 1991), 5.

27. Gail Steketee and Teresa A. Pigott, *Obsessive Compulsive Disorder: The Latest Assessment and Treatment Strategies* (Kansas City, MO: Compact Clinicals, 1999), 1.

28. *New England Journal of Medicine* 321, no. 8 (1989): 539–41.

29. Hollander, "Obsessive-Compulsive Disorder," 3–6.

30. Ibid., 3.

31. See Allan V. Horwitz and Jerome C. Wakefield, *The Loss of Sadness: How Psychiatry Transformed Normal Sorrow into Depressive Disorder* (New York: Oxford University Press, 2007).

11

Atomic Health, or How The Bomb Altered American Notions of Death

JOSEPH MASCO

What happened to health in the atomic age? If we consider health the absence of illness and thus the opposite of death, the atomic bomb has fundamentally altered, if not totally invalidated, the concept. My dictionary defines health as a "condition of being sound in body, mind, or spirit" involving "freedom from physical disease or pain." I like this idea, even yearn for the simple purity it assumes about bodies and knowledge. But this concept of health is at best nostalgic, representing a dream image from an age long surrendered to modern technology and the nation-state. The atomic bomb has not only produced a new social orientation toward death, it has insinuated itself at the cellular level to challenge the very structure of all living organisms (plant, animal, human) on planet Earth. In order to assess a transformation of life on this scale, we need to understand how the atomic bomb has inverted definitions of health and security, remaking them from positive values into an incremental calculus of death.

Instant mass death, individualized cellular mutation, and radiation-induced disease have become normalized threats in our world, producing a new concept of the healthy life as well as a new relationship between citizens and the state mediated by catastrophic risk. The inability to think beyond these atomic potentialities—let alone to reduce the technological, political, and environmental conditions that continue to support them—renders these nuclear effects invisible, normalized, routine. In the atomic age, incipient death has become a form of health itself, both normalized and rendered invisible as a new form of nature. Health, in my formulation, is thus a social construct that regularizes certain potentialities for the human body through an increasingly perverse process of naturalization and amnesia. I propose to track the profound physical and psychological effects of the atomic bomb on American society by exploring how the long-standing state concern with "hygiene" as a joint project of public health and security mutated during the Cold War arms race.

After the atomic bombing of Hiroshima and Nagasaki in August 1945, the technological potential for nuclear war expanded exponentially in the United States, quickly producing a world in which American life could end at any minute. Always on alert, intercontinental missiles, nuclear submarines, and long-range bombers insure that nuclear war can begin any second of the day and, in the first minute of conflict, exceed the total destructive power unleashed in all of World War II. The Cold War state installed this new form of total destruction within the minute-to-minute reality of everyday life by calling it "national security." The technological capability for a totalizing mass death has not changed since the dissolution of the Soviet Union and the formal end of the Cold War. It remains a brute fact of the life that we live, and have lived for several generations, that our everyday space is imbued with the potential for an unprecedented form of collective death. It is unhealthy to say the very least.

But a radically foreshortened social future is only one possible effect of the nuclear revolution; the other is individualized, covert, unpredictable, and cellular. The atmospheric effects of nuclear development—there have been thousands of nuclear explosions conducted in test sites around the world—delivered vast amounts of radioactive material into the global biosphere. Taken up by global wind currents as well as plants and animals, these materials were delivered into each and every person on the planet and deposited in varying amounts within their genomes. As a result, all of us carry in our bodies traces of Strontium-90 and other human-made radioactive elements from the nuclear test program, making life on planet Earth quite literally a post-nuclear formation.[1]

We don't really talk about atomic health anymore. We reject the domestic costs of the U.S. nuclear project in favor of the more generic discourse of "terrorism" and "WMDs." These terms project responsibility for nuclear fear outward onto often nameless and faceless others. They deny that the United States has been the global innovator in nuclear weapons, responsible for every significant technological escalation of the form. The United States also remains the only country to have used nuclear weapons in war, and, in terms of its nuclear development program, it remains the most nuclear-bombed country on Earth (with 904 detonations at the Nevada Test Site alone). Indeed, the social process of coming to terms with an imminent fiery death or a slower, cancerous one has now been normalized as a fact of everyday American life. The roots of nuclear anxiety, however, have not dissipated over time but rather have become more deeply woven into American culture and individual psyches.[2] Whether we choose to recognize it or not, each of us is now a post-nuclear creature, living in a social, biological, and emotional world structured by the cumulative effects of U.S. nuclear weapons science.[3]

If you don't believe me, if you resist my definition of nuclear health as incipient death as absurd or extreme or simply too depressing, consider the hyper-rationalist argument about radioactive life presented by Herman Kahn in his 1960 treatise, *On Thermonuclear War*. Writing as a RAND Corporation strategist, Kahn was influential in conceptualizing U.S. nuclear policy in the early Cold War period. He set out to "think the unthinkable" and work through the details of a nuclear conflict in his book, taking readers from the first salvo of atomic bombs through the collapse of the nation-state and into the possible forms of social recovery.[4] Kahn was a central inspiration for the character of Dr. Strangelove in Stanley Kubrick's 1964 film of the same name, and like the character in the film, he delighted in the shock effects he produced in his audience by exploring the details of nuclear conflict and the conditions of a post-nuclear society.[5] On a surface level, *On Thermonuclear War* is an effort to calculate via cost-benefit analysis the economic, environmental, and health effects of different types of nuclear war. The text, however, also reveals the absurd biological and social stakes of Cold War "national security," calling into question the very "rationality" of the nuclear state. Kahn begins by breaking nuclear war into eight stages. He then assesses the resulting "tragic but distinguishable postwar states" of nuclear conflict depending on the specific war strategy and scale of the conflict.[6] For Kahn, nuclear war is a universe of physical, emotional, and social misery in which decisions still have to be made with stark consequences at each stage of the conflict, from military strategy to medical mobilization and economic recovery. To those who would reject this line of thinking as immoral or perverse, Kahn simply asks: Would you prefer a "post-nuclear America" with 50 million dead or 100 million dead? How about environmental ruin lasting ten years or fifty?[7] Nuclear conflict is rationalized here, as are its vast range of effects, in order to open up a new possibility for post-nuclear governance. Kahn ultimately runs the gruesome numbers to assess the degree of suffering Americans should be willing to accept in order to fight the Cold War. He also attempts to calculate the precise point at which the nuclear destruction would be so great that the "the survivors would envy the dead," thus rendering the Cold War null and void as a collective project (see figure 11.1).[8]

In making these calculations, Kahn provides a new vocabulary of collective risk as well as a variety of new metrics for assessing health in the nuclear age. Consider just the figure titles he uses to illustrate the con-

◆◆◆

TABLE 3
TRAGIC BUT DISTINGUISHABLE POSTWAR STATES

Dead	Economic Recuperation
2,000,000	1 year
5,000,000	2 years
10,000,000	5 years
20,000,000	10 years
40,000,000	20 years
80,000,000	50 years
160,000,000	100 years

Will the survivors envy the dead?

◆◆◆

Figure 11.1. Table from Herman Kahn's *On Thermonuclear War*.

sequences of different nuclear scenarios: "Acceptability of Risks," "Genetic Assumptions," "The Strontium-90 Problem," "Radioactive Environment 100 Years Later," "Morbidity of Acute Total Body Radiation," "Life Shortening," and "Seven Optimistic Assumptions." While these tables detail a scale of suffering that is unprecedented in human experience, Kahn's ultimate metric is not radiation exposure rates or "life shortening" effects or the economic cost of rebuilding destroyed cities and infrastructure, but a rather new kind of social calculus: the "defective child." Acknowledging that the nuclear test programs of the United States and Soviet Union had distributed vast amounts of Strontium-90 in the form of fallout into the global biosphere, Kahn assesses the damage to the human genome. Recognizing that the health effects of Strontium-90 contamination can be both immediate (cancer) and multigenerational (genetic damage), Kahn calculates how many American children will be born severely disabled because of U.S. investment in the atomic bomb. This is a remarkable moment in American history as it recognizes that "national security"— traditionally a defense of both citizens and the state from outside dangers—has been fundamentally altered in the nuclear age, requiring new forms of internal sacrifice. Kahn, however, goes much, much further in his assessment of the Strontium-90 problem, revealing the new terms of nuclear health in a security state that will consider paying any cost right up to the edge of total annihilation in order to win the Cold War:

I could easily imagine a war in which the average survivor received about 250 roentgens . . . This would mean that about 1 percent of the children who could have been healthy would be defective; in short, the number of children born seriously defective would increase, because of war, to about 25 per cent above the current rate. This would be a large penalty to pay for a war. More horrible still, we might have to continue to pay a similar price for 20 or 30 or 40 generations. But even this is a long way from annihilation. It might well turn out, for example, that U.S. decision makers would be willing, among other things, to accept the high risk of an additional 1 per cent of our children being born deformed if that meant not giving up Europe to Soviet Russia. Or it might be that under certain circumstances the Russians would be willing to accept even higher risk than this, if by doing so they could eliminate the United States.[9]

It might well turn out . . . In a world where a security state can imagine as a viable calculus exchanging the health of its children *in perpetuity* for a political victory, the terms of both "public health" and "security" have been mightily and permanently altered. We have moved from a notion of health as an absence of disease to a graded spectrum of dangerous effects now embedded in everyday life. Health, as Kahn presents it here, is a statistical calculation rather than a lived experience, and it is precisely by approaching health as a population effect rather than an individual one that he creates the appearance of rationality.

Kahn's interest in thinking through nuclear warfare, however, does force him, in a few rare but telling moments, to confront the raw physical reality of the human body. Food, for example, would be a major concern in a postnuclear world, and Kahn imagines nuclear war scenarios in which U.S. agriculture could be "suspended" for fifty to a hundred years.[10] Since nuclear war in the era of thermonuclear weapons would spread its effects over the entire continental United States, Kahn focuses on how to manage food produced in a largely contaminated environment. His answer once again points to a new concept of health as incipient death. He proposes to classify food based on the amount of Strontium-90 contamination it contains in groups labeled "A" (little contamination) to "E" (heavily contaminated), and then to distribute the food based on the following criteria:

The A food would be restricted to children and to pregnant women. The B food would be a high-priced food available to everybody. The C food would be a low-priced food also available to everybody. Finally, the D food would be restricted to people over age forty or fifty. Even though this food would be unacceptable for children, it probably would be acceptable for those past middle age, partly because their bones are already formed so that they do not pick up anywhere near as much strontium as the young, and partly because at these low levels of contamination it generally takes some decades for cancer to develop. Most of these people would die of other causes before they got cancer. Finally there would be an E food restricted to the feeding of animals whose resulting use (meat, draft animals, leather, wool, and so on) would not cause an increase in the human burden of Sr-90.[11]

These people would die before they got cancer. Thus, while contamination is total, linking all Americans in a post-nuclear reality, the role of governance is not to prevent disaster but to minimize its effects through the rational calculation of individual age versus the longevity of radioactive materials in the distribution of food. Again, there is no concept of health here if by health we mean an absence of disease or risk. There is rather the naturalization of a new baseline reality (in this case a very contaminated North America and a damaged human genome) within which to begin anew the calculations of effective medical governance. Specifically, the length of time it takes for cancer to appear is calculated against the expected longevity of middle-aged Americans in a post-nuclear world and thereby eliminated as a concern. Under this line of thinking, it is not a sacrifice if you die before the health effects of eating radioactive food give you a fatal cancer.

Kahn recognizes that the psychology of a post-nuclear world would also be a major source of conflict. His analysis participates in a long-running state concern about how emotions—fear, panic, and terror—influence mass populations at a time of constant crisis. He asks his readers to consider this:

Now just imagine yourself in the postwar situation. Everybody will have been subjected to extremes of anxiety, unfamiliar environment, strange foods, minimum toilet facilities, inadequate shelters and the like. Under these conditions some high percentage of the population is going to become nauseated, and nausea is very catching. If one man vomits, everybody vomits. It would not be surprising if almost everybody vomits. Almost everyone is likely to think he has received too much radiation. Morale may be so affected that many survivors may refuse to participate in constructive activities, but would content themselves with sitting down and waiting to die—some may even become violent and destructive.[12]

If one man vomits, everybody vomits. For Kahn, the question is not how to avoid a world where nuclear war is possible but rather how to help individuals understand the meaning of their own gag reflexes. Thus, he proposes a national program to distribute radiation meters throughout all towns and cities as a means to help survivors determine if their physical responses are acute radiation poisoning, the flu, or merely the correct reaction to a world destroyed. Kahn here moves from nausea to panic as an immediate problem of a post-nuclear world. In doing so, he participates in the chief project of civil defense in the early Cold War period—an emotional adjustment of the American public to the reality of nuclear warfare. Having provided radiation meters, the state can now say that citizens possess the means of self-regulating their emotions in a post-nuclear crisis, thus refocusing the crisis from one of mass casualties and destruction to the issue of how individuals control themselves.

The crucial point here is that Herman Kahn's examination of the effects of nuclear war, though widely read in government circles, did not produce a retreat from the escalating arms race but rather an ongoing project to normalize nuclear war as simply another element of risk in everyday life. The Geiger counter becomes the perfect emblem of this logic as it cannot prevent radiation exposure, only document its occurrence. Put differently, nuclear terror—with all its stomach-turning, mind-wrenching, multitudinous forms of anxiety—was never the enemy during the Cold War; this terror was a core tool of the U.S. security state. U.S. officials did not define mental and physical health during the height of the Cold War as an absence of anxiety or injury but rather as the correct response to it, an emotional self-discipline grounded in normalization rather than abjection or terror.

What kind of governance is this? And what has happened to the idea of public health as a state project devoted to improving the lives of citizens? While nuclear war has not yet occurred on the scale Kahn imagined, the effects of the nuclear test project distributed fallout and other environmental contamination on a massive scale to U.S. citizens. The combined effects of environmental damage and social anxiety created by the nuclear arms race fundamentally altered—indeed, placed in opposition—the concepts of "national security" and "public health." In other words, the U.S. effort to build an atomic bomb did not just create a new kind of weapon; it revolutionized American society. The achievement of the bomb in 1945 certainly transformed the nature of military affairs, but it also fundamentally altered the citizen-state relationship and created a new concept of state power, the nuclear superpower. How does nuclear superpower status change concepts of health in the United States as well as alter the state's commitment to improving the lives of its citizens? It is important to remember that the roughly ten thousand nuclear weapons that the United States maintains in its current arsenal (and the vast means of delivering them via aircraft, submarines, cruise missiles, and intercontinental missiles) are capable of holding the entire planet hostage. The first technological achievement of the Cold War state was the production of a 24/7 system of global surveillance and nuclear war fighting capability. This "closed world" system, as Paul Edwards has described it, has kept the world on the edge of a nuclear conflict that could happen with less than ten minutes of warning.[13] Since there is no interior or exterior to this global logic which makes a claim on every living being on the planet, the bomb does not produce "bare life" (a reduction to a purely biological condition) or a "state of exception" in Giorgio Agamben's formulation;[14] in its totalizing scope and effects, it is something rather new in human history.

The modern state form is grounded, as Michel Foucault has argued, in the management of internal populations and the constant improvement of the means of securing that population from a variety of threats. The state's effort to improve and regulate the lives of citizens in terms of hygiene, disease, mental health, and education not only produced the social sciences but also mobilized state power in ways that touched every citizen—from taxes, to inoculations against disease, to the structure of the school system, to the safety of roads, and to the logics of imprisonment (for crime, insanity, and infectious disease). Modern technology as well as modern social science provided the means for constant social improvement as the nation-state form developed, constructing for citizens an imagined future in which health was to be an endless horizon of better living and part of an increasingly secure world. More state security was thus coterminous with the promise of more security for the individual, in other words, a happier, healthier life. This narrative of idealized "progress" was possible until the atomic revolution, which both underscored the reality of radical technological change and invalidated the state's ability to regulate society at the level of health and happiness. Security and health, which were linked for several hundred years in the development of the modern state concept, became contradictory ideas after 1945, all but invalidated as intellectual concepts when challenged by the nuclear reality of the Cold War.

Foucault seems to acknowledge this in his lectures on security. He notes that something fundamental about the state changes after 1945, disrupting his theory about the evolution of state power from monarchal authority through the modern nation-state form, which relies on a variety of means of influencing individuals (discipline) and populations (biopower) in constituting its power.[15] In *Society Must Be Defended*, he argues:

> The workings of contemporary political power are such that atomic power represents a paradox that is difficult, if not impossible, to get around. The power to manufacture and use the atom bomb represents the deployment of a sovereign power that kills, but it is also the power to kill life itself. So the power that is being exercised in this atomic power is exercised in such a way that it is capable of suppressing life itself. And, therefore, to suppress itself insofar as it is the power that guarantees life. Either it is sovereign and uses the atom bomb, and therefore cannot be power, biopower, or the power to guarantee life, as it has been ever since the nineteenth century. Or, at the opposite extreme you no longer have a sovereign right that is in excess of biopower, but a biopower that is in excess of sovereign right.[16]

The "excess" biopower produced by the bomb is a topic that bears much scrutiny, for the United States has literally built itself through nuclear weaponry. In his *Atomic Audit*, Stephen Schwartz has documented the fact that between 1940 and 1996, the United States spent *at least* $5.8 trillion on nuclear weapons.[17] This makes the bomb the third-largest federal expenditure since 1940, just after non-nuclear military spending and Social Security and accounting for roughly eleven cents out of every federal dollar spent. After the atomic destruction of Hiroshima and Nagasaki, the relationship among military, governmental, industrial, and academic institutions grew as these institutions supported a U.S. security state that was founded on nuclear weaponry and anti-communism. The Cold War nuclear standoff consequently became the ground for a new articulation of state power as well as a new social contract in the United States, transforming the terms of everyday life as well as the very definition of public health.

The atomic revolution, however, presented an immediate contradiction to U.S. policymakers about how to define security and health. By the early 1950s, it was clear that the atomic test program in the Pacific was distributing fallout globally even as the expanding arms race with the Soviet Union made possible the extinction of both nation-states and whole ecosystems. Similarly, the decision to open a continental test site in Nevada in 1951 (to lower the costs of nuclear weapons research) insured the direct exposure of Americans with each and every above-ground detonation. Figure 11.2 is a National Cancer Institute county-by-county map of Iodine-131 contamination from above-ground nuclear testing in the United States. Similar contamination maps could be drawn for Strontium-90, Cesium-137, Plutonium-237, and other radionuclides.

The construction of a new national security apparatus, which attacked public health with each detonation, thus required a new kind of collective sacrifice. Not able to pursue both the atomic bomb and the protection of citizens (in the classic sense of not exposing them to damaging health effects), the United States chose instead to normalize the nuclear crisis as a new form of nature. In effect, the Cold War state minimized the health effects of the atomic test program while constantly inflating fears of a Soviet attack in order to create a perception-based form of risk management. It then told citizens that the central problem of the nuclear age was just in their heads. Nuclear war was officially converted into a question of emotional self-control.

In other words, mental health was increasingly fused with national security after 1945 as the United States mobilized nuclear logics to remake its social institutions and its approach to global affairs. Nuclear fear, a unique physiological and mental state first achieved via the atomic bombing of Hiroshima and Nagasaki, quickly became the basis for a permanent wartime economy in the United States and the total mobilization of American political, scientific, academic, and military institutions. With the first Soviet nuclear detonation in 1949, the United States became a paranoid state, seeing communists and nuclear threats everywhere at home and around the world. The nuclear project not only coordinated American institutions in support of a military agenda, it enabled a vision of the entire world as defensible, vulnerable space. "Containing communism" around the world placed U.S. citizens in a new relationship to the security state, which required not only unprecedented financial commitments during "peacetime" but also a parallel project to transform Americans into Cold Warriors. For U.S. policy makers, an immediate question was how to avoid creating an apathetic public on the one hand or a terrorized one on the other—how to create public support for an unprecedented, and potentially unending, militarism.[18]

At the height of the Cold War emotional management project, a new form of mental health practice materialized. As Jonathan Metzl has documented, the nuclear crisis of the mid-1950s was coterminous with the discovery and first mass-marketing of antidepressants in the United States.[19] Psychopharmacology produced a revolution in the very idea of mental health as individuals could now regulate their brain chemistry in an effort to achieve a state of internal calm. Metzl shows how the arrival of psychopharmaceuticals immediately began to replace psychotherapy as the dominant paradigm in treating mental illness. Thus, psychotherapy moved away from personal history and

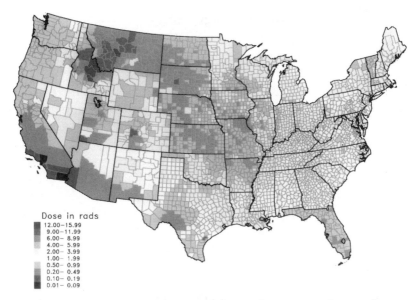

Per capita thyroid doses resulting from
all exposure routes from all tests

Dose in rads
12.00−15.99
9.00−11.99
6.00− 8.99
4.00− 5.99
2.00− 3.99
1.00− 1.99
0.50− 0.99
0.20− 0.49
0.10− 0.19
0.01− 0.09

Figure 11.2. National Cancer Institute Map of Iodine-131 Contamination from Nuclear Tests in Nevada (Courtesy National Cancer Institute).

trauma as an explanatory mode for mental illness at precisely the moment in which trauma was both nationalized and codified within the Cold War system. By eliminating history and experience as an explanatory mechanism, mental treatment could be re-imagined as solely a chemical negotiation, not one involving the social contradictions produced by a nuclear arms race. And by calibrating their emotions to the expectations of Cold War society through drugs, many Americans moved closer to normalizing a state of emergency in everyday life. Anxiety, however, was both a resource and a problem for the early Cold War state.

For the architects of the Cold War system within the Truman and Eisenhower administrations, the solution to public mobilization was a new kind of project, one pursued with help from social scientists and the advertising industry, to teach citizens a specific kind of cognitive and emotional attitude toward the bomb. Drawing on the historic concept of defense as a protection of citizens, the federal program for "civil defense" was actually a quite radical effort to psychologically and emotionally remake Americans

as Cold Warriors. It turned the idea of public protection—a classic definition of security—into a mental operation, concerned almost exclusively with
perceptions, emotions, and self-discipline. This project took the form of an
elaborate propaganda campaign involving films, literature, town meetings,
and educational programs designed to teach Americans to fear the bomb;
to define and limit that nuclear fear in ways useful to the Cold War project;
and to move responsibility for domestic nuclear crisis from the state to citizens, enabling all citizens to have a role in a new collective form of American militarism. Through the 1950s, Civil Defense involved yearly simulations
of nuclear attacks on the United States, in which designated American cities would act out nuclear catastrophe. Local newspapers would run banner
headlines—"Washington DC, Detroit Destroyed by Hydrogen Bombs"—·
allowing civic leaders and politicians to lead theatrical evacuations of the city
that were filmed by television cameras.[20] The formal goal of this state program was to transform "nuclear terror," which was interpreted by officials as
a paralyzing emotion, into "nuclear fear," an affective state that would allow
citizens to function in a time of crisis. As Guy Oaks has documented in *The
Imaginary War*, civil defense programs of the 1950s and '60s sought to do
nothing less than "emotionally manage" U.S. citizens through nuclear fear.[21]

Moreover, since the Cold War was recognized as a state of long-term crisis, civil defense was designed to create a new kind of citizen equipped with a
psychological and emotional constitution capable of negotiating the day-to-
day, minute-to-minute nuclear threat for the long haul. In addition to turning the domestic space of the home into the front line of the Cold War, civil
defense argued that citizens should be psychologically prepared every second
of the day to deal with a potential nuclear attack. Thus, the Cold War state
gave up on the idea of merely preventing attack (part of the traditional logic
of security), and via the discourse of civil defense, demanded that citizens
accept personal responsibility for surviving nuclear conflict. The key move
in this shift from emphasizing protection to vulnerability in public safety
was a campaign to make panic—not nuclear war—the official enemy. As Val
Peterson, the first head of the Federal Civil Defense Administration (FCDA),
wrote in 1953:

> Ninety per cent of all emergency measures after an atomic blast will
> depend on the prevention of panic among the survivors in the first 90 sec-
> onds. Like the A-bomb, panic is fissionable. It can produce a chain reaction
> more deeply destructive than any explosive known. If there is an ultimate
> weapon, it may well be mass panic—not the A-bomb.[22]

PANIC STOPPERS
How to keep from being a victim of panic

Face the Facts — The more you learn, the safer you are. Insulate yourself against panic by finding out all you can about the enemy's weapons — A-bombs, germ and gas warfare, sabotage and rumor war. Misinformation and lack of information breed panic.

Get Ready at Home — Preparedness is good preventive medicine against panic. Prepare and train your family so that the members can perform their duties like trained soldiers under fire. Here's how:

1. Talk to your family about the dangers you face. Work out practice drills so you all know what to do—at home, at work or at school.

2. Get a civil defense emergency first-aid kit together and learn how to use it.

3. Put away a three-day emergency supply of food and water—enough to take care of the whole family and its special needs.

4. Build a home shelter if you live near a target area. If you can't build one, pick out the safest shelter area in your home. Personal shelter can help save your life.

5. Be sure you have a workable AM Radio, preferably battery-operated, in your shelter area. Remember the Conelrad frequencies—640 and 1240—where in an emergency you can get official news and civil defense instructions.

6. Take a Red Cross first-aid course as soon as possible. In the meantime, study the civil defense booklet, Emergency Action to Save Lives. You can get it at your local defense office or at the Government Printing Office, Washington 25, D.C. It costs five cents.

7. Practice fireproof housekeeping; learn how to fight small fires in your home before they can become big ones. There's a nickel government manual for that, too: Fire-Fighting for Householders.

8. Learn the simple steps your family should take to protect themselves against germ warfare. That calls for one more government pamphlet: What You Should Know about Biological Warfare. Cost: 10 cents.

Get Leadership Training — Invest a few hours a week in basic training for one of the organized civil defense services so that you will be ready for group action in any emergency.

Make Fear Work For You — Don't be ashamed of being scared. If an attack comes, you will be scared and so will everyone else. It is *what you do* when you are afraid that counts. Fear can be healthy if you know how to use it; it can make you more alert and stronger at a time when you and your neighbors must act to protect yourselves.

Spike That Rumor — Don't swallow everything you hear. Recognize wartime rumor and gossip for what they are—enemy weapons of the most dangerous kind. Don't let the enemy play you for a sucker — don't pass on rumors. Check any story you hear. Make sure that the facts are from official sources before you repeat them.

Figure 11.3. Chart from Val Peterson's "Panic: The Ultimate Weapon?" (Federal Civil Defense Administration).

Panic is fissionable. Indeed, Peterson not only argued that Americans were particularly "susceptible to panic" but offered a checklist on how citizens could become "panic stoppers" by training themselves for nuclear attack and becoming like "soldiers" at home (see figure 11.3).

Thus, the official message from the early Cold War state was that self-control was the best way for citizens to fight a nuclear war, revealing a national project to both colonize and normalize everyday life with nuclear fear. Panic, as Jackie Orr has so powerfully shown, became more than a means of managing populations in the nuclear age. It remade the individual as a permanently insecure node in the larger Cold War system.[23] Regulating the psychology of a nation-state at this level, however, demanded that Cold War policymakers understand how to produce panic as well as calm it. As Orr has argued, this effort produced a collapsing field of mental health, national security, and individualized identity formation across the frontiers of gender, family, expertise, and self-knowledge.[24] The U.S.

nuclear project writ large required citizens to accept as normal social conditions that were both pathologically insecure and intellectually irreconcilable with health.

The FCDA effort to regulate the national public via images of nuclear conflict took on extraordinary proportions, involving massive, public exercises in which citizens acted out their own destruction and where the state set out to show citizens what a post-nuclear world might look like.[25] The Cold War security state ultimately sought to use nuclear fear to promote a new kind of social and psychological hygiene, one uniquely suited for a nuclear age. In the 1954 FCDA film, *The House in the Middle*, for example, we see that nuclear fear could be harnessed to any kind of domestic project, including household cleanliness (see figure 11.4).

Presented as an atomic experiment, the film documents how nuclear flash, heat, and blast effects engage model houses built at the Nevada Test Site. The three houses presented in the film are in different stages of cleanliness and repair and filmed against the stark desert landscape. The narrator offers this description of the project:

> Three identical miniature frame houses, with varying exterior conditions, all the same distance from the point of the explosion. The house on the right, an eyesore. But you've seen these same conditions in your own hometown: old unpainted wood, and look at the paper, leaves and trash in the yard. In a moment, you'll see the results of atomic heat flash on this house: the house on the left. Typical of many homes across the nation: heavily weathered, dry wood, in run-down condition. This house is the product of years of neglect. It has not been painted regularly. It is dry and rotten—a tinderbox ready to turn into a blazing torch. The house in the middle: in good condition, with a clean, unlittered yard. The exterior has been painted with ordinary, good quality house paint. Light painted surfaces reflect heat and the paint also protects the wood from weathering and water damage. Let's see what happens under atomic heat.[26]

The moralizing tone of the narration underscores that this film is ultimately an effort to recuperate the classic definition of hygiene as a social responsibility, and in so doing to create an image of a state that treats nuclear crisis as it would an infectious disease or a natural disaster. The centerpiece of the film is the slow-motion footage of the atomic blast wave hitting the model houses. The houses on the right and left ignite and burn to the ground, leav-

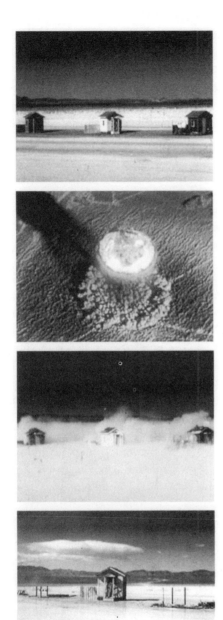

Figure 11.4. Stills from
The House in the Middle
(Federal Civil Defense
Administration).

ing the house in the middle standing. After contemplating this slow-motion destruction in detail, the narrator reexamines the ashes of the houses on the right and left and asks against somber background music, "Which of these is your house? This one? The house on the right? Dilapidated with paper, dead grass, litter everywhere? The house on the left—unpainted, run-down, neglected? Is this your house?" Then on an upbeat music cue, the narrator concludes:

> The house in the middle—cleaned up, painted up, and fixed up, exposed to the same searing atomic heat wave—did not catch fire. Close inspection reveals only a slight charring of the painted outer surface. Yes, the white house in the middle survived an atomic heat flash. These civil defense tests prove how important upkeep is to our houses and town.[27]

Only a slight charring. Household cleanliness is directly linked here to the likelihood of winning or losing a nuclear war. Hygiene, as a classic domain of state intervention into public health, is remade as a means of surviving not illness but nuclear attack. Indeed, the film does not mention fallout or radiation effects at all. The implicit message of the film is that each citizen should patrol his or her neighborhood for trash and feel free to discipline neighbors into perfect home performances. *The House in the Middle* argues ultimately that appearances are more important than reality, that a fresh coat of paint is more important than recognizing the city-killing power of nuclear weapons. Indeed, it offers citizens the opportunity to manically tend to their homes in every detail, from paint and yard work to furnishings and foodstuffs, as a means of achieving public health and national security, even as the reality of thermonuclear warfare promises little to no hope of survival.

The House in the Middle demonstrates how the terms of everyday life in the first decades of the Cold War were saturated with a new kind of state discourse, one that used nuclear fear to promote its policies. The challenge in such a psychological strategy, of course, is one of modulation—enough fear to produce support for U.S. Cold War policies, but not too much to generate a counter-movement. Indeed, the debates about nuclear fallout and the ineffectual nature of the Civil Defense program eventually forced the nuclear program into a major reorganization in the early 1960s. Civil defense, at this time, was factually wrong in many of its claims about the ability to survive a nuclear war. Moreover, the effort by Herman Kahn and others to "think the unthinkable" revealed to many the impossibility of civil defense in the thermonuclear age. U.S. scientists also produced a powerful anti-nuclear counter-discourse that emphasized the health effects of nuclear testing as well as the false claims of civil defense, challenging the state to return to concepts of security and health committed to improving living conditions rather than normalizing nuclear crisis. But the first decade of the Cold War witnessed the development of an entirely new form of governance, one in which a very public "national security" discourse was used strategically by the state to both mask and enable a global vision grounded in the sacrifice of citizens born and unborn. Public health, in this context, became secondary to a vision of national security that installed new forms of individual death within a larger structure of mass death. The social consequences of the nuclear arms race ultimately inverted the concept of health as absence of disease, replacing it with an increasingly naturalized vision of health as incipient death.

The effects of this joint transformation in the logics of health and national security are still with us today. The reactions to the suicide attacks on Washington, DC and New York in 2001 reinvigorated the emotional management strategy and returned Americans to the logics of survival and sacrifice that structured the Cold War period. The threat of terrorism was, in fact, magnified by the George W. Bush administration into grounds for a fundamental rethinking of U.S. global ambitions as well as U.S. domestic policy, just as the first Soviet nuclear test in 1949 was mobilized by the Truman and Eisenhower administrations to construct the Cold War state. The state's appeal to citizens after 2001 was also modeled on the early civil defense campaigns as it argued for a normalization rather than an elimination of a totalized threat. Consider, for a moment, the first round of civil defense advertisements by the newly formed Department of Homeland Security in 2003 (see figure 11.5).

One commercial begins as a young girl starts working her way across the monkey bars at a playground. Halfway through she stops; while hanging on the bars, she looks directly at the camera and recites the following list: "Batteries, a first-aid kit, enough water for three days, a flashlight, transistor radio, a whistle, a dust mask, a plan." As she exits the apparatus, text flows on to the screen, stating:

BE PREPARED
READY.GOV

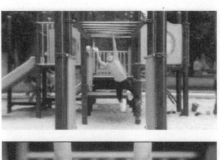

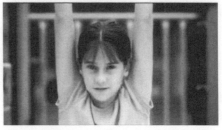

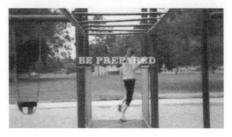

Figure 11.5. Stills from 2003 "America Prepared" Commercial (Department of Homeland Security).

In a second DHS civil defense commercial, a little league baseball game is under way, and mid-pitch the pitcher and batter stop to trade preparedness info (see figure 11.6):

PITCHER: My dad's work number: 212-327-1845.
HITTER: My aunt Judy: 281-837-4066.
PITCHER: A meeting place.
HITTER: A plan.

BE PREPARED
READY.GOV

Fifty years after Val Peterson's national campaign to teach citizens to fear panic more than the bomb, the official position is still that every second of

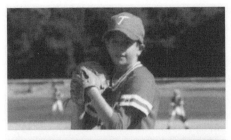

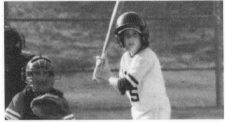

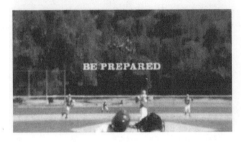

Figure 11.6. Stills from 2003 "America Prepared" Commercial (Department of Homeland Security).

your life should be spent rehearsing the possibility of disaster, training yourself as a citizen to take responsibility for events that are by definition out of your control. Repeating the civil defense logics from the first decades of the Cold War, the state is absent here except in its desire to install a specific kind of fear within everyday life through advertising. The first ninety seconds of a crisis are still the most important, requiring that children be prepared to recite emergency information between swings of a little league bat or rungs on the jungle gym. These commercials reiterate the lessons of nuclear civil defense, that everyday life is structured around the possibility of mass injury from one moment to the next and that citizens must take responsibility for their own survival.

One of the most difficult cultural logics to assess is the arrival of a new social relationship to death. The vulnerability of children is one immediate register of American ideas of death, whether revealed in Herman Kahn's meditations on the number of "defective children" it will take to win the Cold War or in these DHS commercials that portray children as robots, preprogrammed to respond to crisis, rehearsing their life-line phone numbers even in the midst of play. Since 1945, the United States has built its national community via contemplation of specific images of mass death while building a defense complex that demands ever more personal sacrifice in the name of security. Health as an absence of disease or anxiety is long gone. What we have instead is a negotiation of degrees of contamination, of degrees of anxious association, of degrees of escalating risk. The initial concept of public health as a key coordinate of the modern state system has been replaced by a governmental calculus based on individual sacrifice. A "war on terror" requires that Americans once again naturalize a notion of health as incipient death, inviting each and every citizen to dust off the familiar logics of Cold War sacrifice and embrace the further collapse of mental health into national security. Demilitarizing the mind by rejecting the "war on terror" project thus contains revolutionary potential; it might finally overthrow a national security project that both relies on and installs ever more deeply the possibility of violence and death into everyday life. In the twenty-first century, the last thing we need is more "health." Demilitarizing the mind, body, and spirit of American citizens by getting rid of the bomb, however, might just open up an entirely new kind of nature—post-national security, post-terror. Panic should be the least of our concerns.

NOTES

1. See Joseph Masco, *The Nuclear Borderlands: The Manhattan Project in Post–Cold War New Mexico* (Princeton: Princeton University Press, 2006), and Arjun Makhijani and Stephen I. Schwartz, "Victims of the Bomb," in *Atomic Audit: The Costs and Consequences of U.S. Nuclear Weapons Since 1940*, ed. Stephen I. Schwartz (Washington, DC: Brookings Institution Press, 1998).

2. See Amy Kaplan, "Homeland Insecurities: Some Reflections on Language and Space," *Radical History Review* 85 (Winter 2003): 82–93.

3. See Masco, "Mutant Ecologies: Radioactive Life in Post-Cold War New Mexico," *Cultural Anthropology* 19, no. 4 (November 2004): 517–50.

4. Herman Kahn, *On Thermonuclear War* (Princeton: Princeton University Press, 1960).

5. See Sharon Ghamari-Tabrizi, *The Worlds of Herman Kahn: The Intuitive Science of Thermonuclear War* (Cambridge, MA: Harvard University Press, 2005).

6. Kahn, *On Thermonuclear War*, 34.

7. Ibid., 19.

8. Ibid., 40.

9. Ibid., 46.

10. Ibid., 66.

11. Ibid., 66–7.

12. Ibid., 86.

13. See Paul N. Edwards, *The Closed World: Computers and the Politics of Discourse in Cold War America* (Cambridge, MA: MIT Press, 1996).

14. See Giorgio Agamben, *Homo Sacer: Sovereign Power and Bare Life* (Stanford: Stanford University Press, 1998).

15. See Michel Foucault, "The Risks of Security," in *Power: Essential Works of Foucault, 1954–1984*, volume III, ed. James Faubion (New York: New Press, 2000), 365.

16. Foucault, *Society Must Be Defended: Lectures at the College de France, 1975–76*, ed. Mauro Bertani and Alessandro Fontana (New York: Picador, 2003), 253.

17. Schwartz, *Atomic Audit*, 1.

18. See Guy Oakes, *The Imaginary War: Civil Defense and American Cold War Culture* (New York: Oxford University Press, 1994), 34.

19. Jonathan Metzl, *Prozac on the Couch: Prescribing Gender in the Era of Wonder Drugs* (Durham: Duke University Press, 2003).

20. See Stacy C. Davis, *Stages of Emergency: Cold War Nuclear Civil Defense* (Durham: Duke University Press, 2007), and Laura McEnaney, *Civil Defense Begins at Home: Militarization Meets Everyday Life in the Fifties* (Princeton: Princeton University Press, 2000).

21. Oaks, *Imaginary War*, 47.

22. Val Peterson, "Panic: The Ultimate Weapon?" Collier's: *The National Weekly*, August 21, 1953, 99.

23. Jackie Orr, *Panic Diaries: A Genealogy of Panic Disorder* (Durham: Duke University Press, 2006), 14.

24. Ibid.

25. See Masco, "Survival Is Your Business: Engineering Ruins and Affect in Nuclear America," *Cultural Anthropology* 23, no. 2 (May 2008): 361–98.

26. Federal Civil Defense Administration, *The House in the Middle*, 1954, 12 min., film.

27. Ibid.

Part IV

Pleasure and Pain after Health

12

How Much Sex Is Healthy?

The Pleasures of Asexuality

EUNJUNG KIM

Physicians, public health practitioners, and "pro-sex" activists may agree that sexual drive is a natural, healthy, and essential aspect of the human. Health risks related to sexual activities are often highlighted by these individuals, but the idea that willingness and capability to have sex reflects and promotes a person's psychological and physiological health is widespread in Western contemporary culture. A popular news Website proclaims, "Want to get healthy? Have sex."[1] A *Newsweek* article elaborates, "Sex is good for adults. Indulging on a regular basis—at least once a week—is even better."[2] The health benefits of sex listed are increased immune strength in fighting off cold and flu, looking younger, burning calories, decreasing women's urinary incontinence, and reducing pain. While expressions of sexuality are regulated in society, the absence of sexual desires, feelings, and activities is seen as abnormal and reflective of poor health because of the explicit connection made between sexual activeness and healthiness. The way we understand desire and the relationship between sex and health are rarely simple. There lies the complexity of the cultural and social dimensions of sex beyond behavior, biological basis, sexual disorder, abstinence, religion, pleasure, and risk.

The public emergence of asexual people in the U.S., U.K., and Canadian media and in global online communities illustrates that some individuals understand their absence of sexual desire as an asexual identity or orientation, not as lack or dysfunction.[3] The Asexual Visibility and Education Network (AVEN) describes an asexual person as someone who does not experience sexual attraction. Some asexual people may experience sexual desire but do not desire to engage with others sexually or desire only to engage in autoerotic practices. Others claim that they are born without sexual feelings entirely and never feel any kind of sexual desire.[4] AVEN asserts on its Website that "Asexuality is not a dysfunction, and there is no need to find a 'cause' or 'cure.'" A *New Scientist* article, "Glad to Be A," explains that some asexuals might simply have extremely low sex drives despite romantic orientation toward males or females. Other asexuals might be attracted to neither gender while they experience their sex drives. Kristin Scherrer, the author of several articles on asexual identity, adds that individuals who identify as asexual may also identify as lesbian, gay, bisexual, transsexual, queer, or heterosexual in their romantic orientation.[5] Many narratives of individuals demonstrate that asexuality escapes monolithic definition, simple behavior patterns, bodily characteristics, and identities despite some researchers' efforts to draw a clear boundary for the "condition." In other words, individuals who identify as asexual vary greatly in their explorations of identity to make sense of themselves as people who have other kinds of orientation outside of the sexual realm. For these reasons, my use of the term "asexuality" is meant to be broad and relatively and subjectively defined as an insufficient or absent willingness to engage in sexual activity with others. This descriptive and relative determination of asexuality is based on cultural assessments of "normal" frequency and level of desire.

Participants in asexual identity movements emphasize that their asexuality is not a problem in their experience and that they are healthy and happy.[6] They also argue that it is mainstream society that denies the existence of asexuality, marginalizes it, and stigmatizes it, and for that reason they are alienated and not recognized for who they are. I argue in this chapter that medical explanations of asexuality as an abnormality that has to be corrected constitute a large part of the stigmatization and marginalization experienced by asexual people. However, the way that asexual activists use the claim of "being healthy" and seek legitimacy and normality in the name of health to counter the pathological charge significantly limits our understandings of diverse asexual lives. By closely analyzing two cultural texts that represent asexual lives from contrasting paradigms, I discuss how asexuality brings new ways of experiencing and understanding pleasure when considered outside of the framework of health and normality. This is not to say that all sexual or asexual practices are completely unrelated to one's health status and bodily events. However, health information and interpretations about sex are grounded too much in belief in universal sexual desire and give too much authority to health professionals to produce "cures" marketed by the sex therapy and pharmaceutical industries. Often, information about sexuality and health is equivocal, incoherent, and politically charged. I am "against health" as it is utilized by medical authorities to determine what is normal and to guard their professional territory, therefore shutting down new and creative understandings about how we might live with or without sex.

Against Pathology, Against Fighting Stigma in the Name of Health

I bring asexuality under the discussion of "against health" for two reasons. First, while sexual practices are heavily regulated in the United States in relation to gender, race, ethnicity, class, ability/disability status, religion, sexual orientation, and age, asexuality is subject to a pathologizing framework that demands a "cure" and "help" under the premise that sexual desire is universally and constantly present in adult life and that its absence reflects pathology or causes harm. As the AVEN Website explains, "In a world where sexuality is promoted as the norm, many asexuals grow up thinking that they're somehow sick, broken, or deficient." Absence of sexual desire may be alterable or not; it may coexist with physiological or psychological conditions; it may be present without any identifiable causes. Labeling all kinds of asexuality as ill-health obscures the diverse and ordinary aspects of asexual experience. According to Leonore Tiefer, the medical and pharmaceutical industries have taken an increasing interest in sex, using various strategies to create a disease of sexual inadequacy through which to market drug treatments.[7] This combination of medicalization of sexuality and market forces promotes the drive for a cure for asexuality. Medical diagnoses associated with asexuality such as Hypoactive Sexual Desire Disorder or Female Sexual Dysfunction may legitimize bodily difficulties that individuals experience as valid signs or serious causes of distress and interpersonal difficulties, but the medical model comes with a cost, solidifying norms and excluding other bodies that do not fit as exceptional and deviant.[8] In fact, distress and relationship difficulties may be caused by external factors such as social pressure, partner expectations, dominant gender role expectations, and stigma. Tiefer also claims that the medical model itself is severely limited in its ability to deal with problems of sexuality because of its separation between mind and body, its biological reductionism, its focus on disease rather than people as a whole, and its reliance on norms. She claims pharmacological research often oversimplifies the sexual difficulties of both men and women because it "promotes genital function as the centrepiece of sexuality and ignores everything else."[9] She further asserts that sexual life has become vulnerable to "disease mongering" because a long history of social and political control of sexual expression has created reservoirs of shame and ignorance, and popular culture has greatly inflated public expectations about sexual function and understandings of the importance of sex to personal and relationship satisfaction.[10]

Second, pathologizing asexuality puts asexual people on the defensive and leads them and some within the media to insist on their normality by using the language of their critics. Some asexual men emphasize the fact that their "plumbing works fine" in response to suspicious inquiries about their underlying problems which include physical abnormality, impotence, or lack of masculinity. Some asexuals argue that they are as normal as sexual persons except they do not desire to have sex with others. A reporter at *New Scientist* who interviewed a leading figure in the asexuality movement felt compelled to reassure readers that the asexual man was nonetheless physically attractive. The reporter describes the man's appearance and then concludes, "He is living proof that it is absolutely wrong to assume asexuals shun sex simply because they can't get any."[11] The seeming normalcy and healthiness of an asexual person operates as an entry toward public acceptance of asexuality. Although correcting the stereotypical image of an asexual person as undesirable or deviant by presenting the relevant "facts" is the goal of such endeavor, it is equally important to remember that being sexually desirable or healthy does not automatically lead to the recognition of asexuality as a legitimate difference. Just as with any other identity group with a significant range of diversity, many members of asexual communities acknowledge that they deal with various health issues as well as mental, physical, and psychological differences, some more common than others. The diversity within asexual groups makes the health claim of asexuality in order to fight pathologization more complicated. Is the claim that "we are not sick" a distancing strategy that erases other asexual people who have mental or physical illnesses, disabilities, and neurological differences? Claiming positive identity based on good health status and normalcy has the potential to ignore those people with various health issues, sexually related or not. Speaking of sex and its absence in the name of health easily falls into the moral and ableist binary of the *good body* and the *bad body*, and it relies on dominant able-bodied (hetero)sexual sex and gender expectations rather than presenting sex as composed of unpredictable and diverse practices, emotions, and reasons.

This is not to suggest that there is a unitary claim of healthiness and able-bodiedness in the asexuality movement that is employed by all asexual people. According to asexual activist David Jay, it is useful to mold the story of asexuality and health according to the audience at hand. To the general public, he emphasizes that he is happy and healthy, highlighting that asexuality is not correlated with any health issues. He explains that the medical conditions of the asexual individuals are not generally discussed with the press in order to avoid conjecture about possible correlations. To medical professionals, he says that asexuals' healthcare needs are not understood properly in medical communities and he emphasizes the need for more partnership. To the asexual community, he argues that asexuality is not a problem in itself but encourages medical consultation when individuals experience a sudden drop in sexual desire.[12] These maneuvers illustrate the multiple ways in which health is related with asexuality, but at the same time, how one has to notice the presence of the negative connection between them either by emphasizing healthiness or avoiding the topic.

Certainly, asexual people's recourse to identity politics and community-building does raise other important questions. Can one be asexual and claim asexuality as a positive identity within a society that understands asexuality not only as a sign of contempt but also as a naturalized trait for some people? What is it like to be asexual when one is not considered sexual at all or is somehow prohibited from being sexual? Many people are ordered into nonsexual and nonreproductive lives because of their age, disability, health, race, gender, class, or appearance. People in minority groups and those with oppressed sexualities have presented disagreements with the idea of asexuality when it is imposed as a stereotype or a mandate. People with disabilities, for example, dispute asexuality as stigma that denies them their basic right and access to sexual, intimate lives. Some Asian American men in the United States engage in online "anti-asexuality" communities that resist the stereotype of the sexually reserved, emasculated, and effete Asian American male (a stereotype that coexists with the highly sexualized yet submissive image of the Asian American female). This activity effectively erases the space for asexual Asian American men. Asexuality is a typical prejudice applied to older persons and lesbians as well. To take this last example, scholars in the field of female sexuality studies challenge the pejorative connotation of inactive sexuality reflected in the term "lesbian bed death," a supposed "drop-off" in sexual activity in long-term lesbian relationships and alleged lower rates of sexual activity for lesbian couples in general. The stigma represented by the discourse of "lesbian bed death" creates a double bind: lesbians were once assumed to be "sick" when they were having sex, but now, according to some lesbian affirmative therapists, lesbians are "sick" when they are not having sex.[13] The activism of asexual people for recognition and respect of their asexual identity challenges the simplified understanding of asexuality only as a status of oppression, which ignores the presence of asexual people within desexualized groups. The discussion of asexuality should be positioned beyond the good (acceptable) body and the bad (unacceptable and therefore to be fixed) body binary; instead, the conundrum of asexuality invites considerations of multiple contestations among a positive identity politics, a medical framework, and labels of oppressed sexuality produced by desexualization, as well as their overlapping grounds. It is important that these examinations consider the possibilities of utilizing a diversity of health statuses and other differences in race, age, disability, religion, and other sexual orientations as a part of a larger asexual embodiment. Sexual rights and asexual rights are not at odds with each other but part of recognizing the intertwined construction of diversity.

"Under the Hood" and Snow Cake: Two Different Paradigms

Authoritative medical explanations defining normal amounts of sex circulate beyond the clinical setting through the medium of popular cultural representations. First aired in 2005, the episode "Under the Hood," part of the Discovery Channel Canada's documentary series *Sexual Secrets*, offers an example of the contestation between medical authorities and individual narratives over the topic of asexuality and sexual dysfunction. The episode deals with various sexual disorders including so-called persistent sexual arousal syndrome, male erectile dysfunction, female post-partum decrease of sexual desire, and sexual anorexia along with the topic of asexual identities. The documentary presents these presumably unknown sexual problems as serious disorders that cause a lot of suffering. The documentary also introduces sites of medical treatment, such as counseling, exercise, and therapies.

In order to introduce the absence of sexual desire as one of these problems, the film crew asks people in the street about not having sexual desire. "Do you think that's possible?" an interviewer asks. One woman says, "Yeah, I think they are called mothers," pointing out how frequently the absence of sexual desire is experienced by many women. Most people, however, characterize sex as necessary and natural, or as one man puts it, "I think people need to have sex to enjoy life." Another woman says, "I don't know [if] asexuality is a normal thing. I think sexuality is a good thing. I think it's a natural thing. And it's healthy. And it's good to be sexual." Through these interviews, the film sets up asexuality as a topic of public opinion that can be voted up or down.

The asexual individuals who address the audience describe their lack of interest in sex not as a problem but as a difference. The documentary rejects their perspective, interrupting each asexual individual's interview with sexual scenes of heterosexual couples in bed, therefore marking a sharp contrast between what these asexual people are saying and what the documentary presents as natural. The film's doubtful attitude toward asexual identity comes across clearly. After the interview with David Jay, the narrator poses a question. "David says he is perfectly content with his asexuality. But is there a dark side to saying no to sex?" The narrator continues, "Are some asexuals ignoring something traumatic from their pasts and denying their true feelings?"

The film focuses on pathological explanations for asexuality, though it does feature one scientist who presents asexuality as an acceptable variation since asexual people pose no threat to society. The documentary highlights the fact that some asexual people are victims of sexual assault, suffer from post-traumatic stress disorder, or have religious guilt. The narrator says, "Asexuals declare that their lack of desire is normal. But some doctors argue that some asexuals are actually suffering deep emotional turmoil. They argue that being asexual is not a choice made from strength but from intense pain." An expert adds, "I hear people make the statement that 'I don't need sex and I'm not unhappy about it.' But I find them suicidal or they're depressed," thus assuming that these psychological difficulties are rooted in asexuality or are the cause of asexuality. What is problematic is that the film squelches diversity within asexual people, combining those who are untroubled by their asexuality and those who suffer and want to be sexual by conflating the two narratives. Moreover, it assumes that asexuality is not acceptable when it is brought by victimization without considering how individuals experience asexuality. This way, the presentation of asexual people as suffering subjects (exclusively due to asexuality) reframes the asexual identity narrative as a harmful coping mechanism that stands in denial of real "turmoil." It is important not to assume all asexual people are victims. Even if asexual people have been victimized, just as have many sexual people, this does not warrant the understanding of asexuality as a damaged sexuality. Asexual people experience their own struggles, experiment and question their sexual/asexual identity, and may want to come out as asexual and work toward developing senses of pride as asexual people. The film does provide access to asexual people's self-representation and its fluid nature, but goes on to present them as self-deceiving through the eyes of doubtful professionals.

To nail down the idea that asexuality is unnatural, the film makes a connection between sex and food, as if refusal of sex were a refusal of necessary sustenance. The analogy between sex and food defies the message of abstinence campaigns that assume that individuals can control and delay their sexual lives as long as they want with their willpower. "Searching for sex is a primal urge," the narrator claims, "almost as basic as hunting for food." The narrator asks viewers to imagine a life without food or sex, and this analogy leads quickly to the idea of sexual anorexia. Another expert on people who are repulsed by sex claims that "sexual anorexics" starve themselves and are full of self-loathing and hatred, and that, just as anorexic people deny themselves nourishment, sexually anorexic people deny themselves sexual contact.[14] Citing the case of a man who prefers a solitary life, the doctor makes the claim that when a man does not have enough male energy, he fears female energy and sees it as dangerous. Effectively converting fear and avoidance of sex into lack of dominant masculinity, the film once more presents an intimate scene of a man and a woman in bed as the ultimate goal in the healing of pathological asexuality. The repeated use of these types of sexual scenes in the documentary, contrasted with sad-looking, frustrated individuals alone in bed, creates a world divided between the sexual and the asexual. The medicalization of asexuality and the denial of asexual identity by health professionals turn individual bodies into medical facts, even though, as sexual scientists increasingly explain, there is neither evidence of psychic inhibition of libido in such individuals nor an effective treatment for people in a long-term state of asexuality.[15]

The film also presents the search for a medical cure for asexuality at a sexual treatment center in Chicago. The center recommends that women who do not want to have sex with their husbands maintain some kind of sexual relationship with their partner and think of it as a gift to them. Women exercise to increase their ability to orgasm and to fulfill their potential to enjoy sex. When a woman speaks with joy about meeting so many other women who experience no sexual desire, the idea is not that she has found a community to affirm her—an empowering experience shared by asexual people visiting online communities such as AVEN. Rather, the community attests to the severity of her problem. In fact, the documentary describes members of AVEN as another group of patients in need of medical treatment and healing: "An essential element of any healing is asking out loud for help, understanding and hopefully finding a community to share a journey with." The journey of asexual people is, by implication, toward healing and the joy of sex, not toward a different identity and a respected difference.

As asexuality activists oppose the prevailing view that stigmatizes asexuality, their resistance can be assisted by cultural representations of asexuality outside of medically dominated discourse. My second example offers the possibility of resistance necessary to think critically about asexuality outside of the discourse of health and able-bodiedness. *Snow Cake* (2006), by British filmmaker Marc Evans, is a fictional film that depicts asexuality in a quite different way than the documentary "Under the Hood." It raises awareness about autism by focusing on the everyday life of an adult mother with autism living in Canada, but it also features asexuality as a main component of the highly verbal and autistic character's life. The film presents a compelling and vivid setting for asexuality beyond the realm of usual imperatives about asexuality as abnormality. The film's unusual quality comes from its presentation of an asexual woman who is not perfectly "normal" except for being asexual. Together with autism, asexual characteristics can be easily perceived as anti-social and anti-sexual attitudes. However, the film does not apply either moral or medical judgments to the main character. Rather, it depicts asexuality and autism as forms of human diversity and metaphorizes them as endlessly different kinds of snowflakes.

Aloof, middle-aged Englishman Alex Hughes (Alan Rickman) gives a ride to a teenage stranger, Vivienne (Emily Hampshire), who dies instantly when Alex's car is struck by a truck on the road. Mourning Vivienne's death, Alex visits her mother, Linda Freeman (Sigourney Weaver), and finds her actions strikingly non-reactive compared to those of a typical grieving mother. Puzzled by Linda's seeming indifference, Alex asks Linda's neighbor, Maggie (Carrie-Anne Moss), about this behavior, to which Maggie answers that Linda is autistic. To Alex, Linda does not appear to be grieving, especially when she describes the meaning of the death of Vivienne in functional terms of not having someone to carry out the garbage or with whom to have fun. Alex decides to stay with her until garbage day on Linda's request, thus temporarily solving the practical challenge that follows Vivienne's death.

Alex soon learns that Linda is not only autistic but asexual, although the term "asexual" is not used in the film. The next morning Alex discovers Linda lying down in the backyard, eating snow with increasing joy. Linda describes her feeling to Alex by referring to sexual orgasm. "Vivienne once described an orgasm to me," Linda says. "It sounds like an inferior version of what I feel when I have a mouthful of snow." On another occasion, Linda insists that Alex join her on the trampoline, and he jumps up and down while she lies on her back and enjoys the continuous bouncing. The snow-eating and trampoline scenes propose an equivalent to sexual pleasure experienced by the asexual Linda, giving the film a way for sexual and non-autistic audience members to imagine Linda's pleasure. In fact, the film carefully carves out Linda's asexuality to contrast her with her neighbor Maggie's sexual activeness (which also marginalizes her in the conservative community). The film presents the lives of two different women, mediated by the socially distant Alex, as two alternative lifestyles, each with its own hardships and joys. Having had a complicated past, Alex finds comfort in both the social, inquisitive, sexual Maggie and the asocial, indifferent, asexual Linda. Linda's asexuality is a characteristic related to her disability, but not—and this is of critical importance—a pathological condition to be examined. In an emblematic moment, Alex acknowledges the pleasure Linda takes in eating snow by leaving in her freezer a cake made of snow as a good-bye gift, perhaps providing her with the experience of an "orgasm,"[16] while neither problematizing her asexuality nor suggesting that asexuality is a state of deprivation.

The film also uses motherhood as another important reference point to prevent the audience from assuming that Linda's asexuality is either a pathology or an absolute condition caused by her autism. Given Linda's lack of interest in sex, Alex is puzzled as to how Vivienne "happened." Linda's father admits that no one knows the answer. The father tells Alex that he first suspected that the pregnancy was the result of a sexual assault. In fact, disabled women's sexual experience is often assumed to be the product of sexual violence not only because there is a high prevalence of sexual violence in women with disabilities, but also because the popular imagination cannot conceive of disabled women as exercising sexual agency. However, in this case, as her father further explains, Linda refused to answer questions about sexual violence and didn't seem to be upset. Her parents speculate that her pregnancy might have been a result of experimentation with her colleague at the community center. The film carefully avoids scripting the common image of a woman with a disability as an eternal child, an innocent angel, or a victim of sexual violence who needs protection. The film does not give any definite answer about how and why Linda engaged in sexual activity or whether or not she was sexually traumatized. The audience members are directed only to Linda herself and encouraged to move away from the desire to question or probe the apparent mismatch between motherhood and autism with asexuality.

Apart from characteristics unique to their different genres, "Under the Hood" and Snow Cake take thematically different courses in exploring lives without sex. With its authority of medical professionals and its dramatized sexual scenes, "Under the Hood" attempts to frame an exposé about a topic that is completely unknown to its general audience, thereby making asexuality exotic and unfamiliar. It imagines asexuality as a serious sign of health problems—despite its attempt to present asexual people's points of view—and creates hope for its audience when it proposes medical treatment for individuals struggling for a cure. Snow Cake proposes another point of view that does not make health a legitimizing or disapproving tool. It represents the imagined pleasures and heightened sensations of an asexual woman with autism experiencing a great pleasure that comes from other sensual activities.[17]

Conclusion

Medical knowledge about the topics of asexuality and sexuality circulates into public awareness in a way that privileges the professional point of view over individual experiences and their creative interpretations. "The power of medical ideology in the construction of sexual desire derives from its expansion, its authoritative voice," Janice Irvine explains.[18] In addition to medical ideology, Irvine also notes that popular representations associate "problems" of desire with disease, often adopting a language of dysfunction. I offered the text of "Under the Hood" as an example of popular culture's narration of sexual desire through the language of medical dysfunction based on normative gender expectations. Closely reading representations of asexual people with disabilities may be instructive as we look for more nuanced and less prescriptive ways of configuring sexual desire or its absence without erasing its diversity. The pathological framework for asexuality is symptomatic of a larger trend in which sexuality is tied up with the image of "normal" bodies. Understanding asexuality as a disorder that can and must be treated reveals anxiety about unstable aspects of sex, body functions, and sexual desire. By refusing to think about sexuality as a matter of health, I have argued that asexuality brings new ways of experiencing and understanding pleasure.

NOTES

1. Laura Berman, "Want to Get Healthy? Have Sex," *Today*, January 15, 2008, http://www.msnbc.msn.com/id/22650190.

2. Temma Ehrenfeld, "Six Reasons to Have Sex Every Week," *Newsweek*, December 10, 2007, http://www.newsweek.com/id/74575.

3. AVEN: The Asexuality Visibility and Education Network, http://www.asexuality.org.

4. Geraldine Levi Joosten-van Vilsteren, Edmund Fortuin, David Walker, and Christine Stone, *Nonlibidoism: The Short Facts* (Amsterdam: Lavender Publishers, 2005). Although the authors in this collection prefer to use the term "nonlibidoism" and not asexuality, I consider asexuality in a broader sense to include nonlibidoists, or people who are born without any sexual feelings.

5. Kristin Scherrer, "Asexuality: Understanding Sexual Diversities," in *Talk About It: National Coming Out Month Magazine 2007* (Ann Arbor: Office of LGBT Affairs and Division of Student Affairs, University of Michigan, 2007), 22–23.

6. Anonymous, "Is There an Asexual Closet?" Asexuality Visibility and Education Network, http://www.asexuality.org/en/lofiversion/index.php/t8569.html.

7. See Leonore Tiefer, "Female Sexual Dysfunction: A Case Study of Disease Mongering and Activist Resistance," *PLoS Medicine* 3, no. 4 (April 2006): 436–40. Ray Moynihan and Matthew Anderson are also concerned that pharmaceutical companies influenced the creation of female Hypoactive Sexual Desire Disorder (HSDD) as a disease in order to promote testosterone as a treatment. See Ray Moynihan, "The Making of a Disease: Female Sexual Dysfunction," *British Medical Journal* 326, no. 7379 (January 4, 2003): 45–47; "The Marketing of a Disease: Female Sexual Dysfunction," *British Medical Journal* 330, no. 7484 (January 22, 2005): 192–94; and Matthew Anderson, "Is Lack of Sexual Desire a Disease? Is Testosterone the Cure?" *Medscape Ob/Gyn and Women's Health* 10, no. 2 (2005).

8. Some researchers believe that asexuality and the medical diagnosis of HSDD are not the same thing, while others believe that they are undoubtedly connected.

9. Leonore Tiefer, "The Medicalization of Sexuality: Conceptual, Normative, and Professional Issues," *Annual Review of Sex Research* 7 (1996): 252–82.

10. Tiefer, "Female Sexual Dysfunction," 45–47.

11. Sylvia Pagán Westphal, "Glad to Be A," *New Scientist* 184, no. 2469 (October 14, 2004): 38–43.

12. Personal communication with David Jay, March 2009.

13. In order to disprove the asexuality label, some researchers argue that there is not sufficient data about the definition of lesbian sexual behavior itself. They further emphasize that lesbian sexuality is "healthier" and more "intimate" than typical genital activity. See Marny Hall, "Not Tonight Dear, I'm Deconstructing a Headache: Confessions of a Lesbian Sex Therapist," in *A New View of Women's Sexual Problems,* ed. Ellyn Kaschak and Leonore Tiefer (New York: Haworth Press, 2001).

14. Some media outlets present professional opinions of looking at asexuality as normal if it does not cause distress and conflict in a marriage or relationship, but they also quote sex therapists' dismissive attitudes of the legitimacy of asexual identity claims. A recent article in the *New York Times*, for example, quotes Dr. Leonard R. Derogatis as saying that "Sex is a natural drive, as natural as the drive for sustenance and water to survive. It's a little difficult to judge these folks as normal." See Mary Duenwald, "For Them, Just Saying No Is Easy," *New York Times,* June 9, 2005, http://www.nytimes.com/2005/06/09/fashion/thursdaystyles/09asexual.html. Specialists appearing on television also worry that the resort to asexuality identity claims is a self-fulfilling prophecy because asexuals want to ignore real problems and possible treatments. These specialists sometimes refer to asexuals as "sexually neutered." See "Asexuals," *20/20* television program aired on ABC network, September 5, 2006.

15. See Elizabeth K. Ullery, Vaughn S. Millner, and Heath A. Willingham, "The Emergent Care and Treatment of Women with Hypoactive Sexual Desire Disorder," *The Family Journal* 10, no. 3 (July 2002): 349; Helen Singer Kaplan, *The Sexual Desire Disorders: Dysfunctional Regulation of Sexual Motivation* (New York: Brunner/Mazel, 1995), 5; and Sandra R. Leiblum and Raymond C. Rosen, eds., *Sexual Desire Disorders* (New York: Guilford, 1988), 4.

16. Disability studies and film scholar Sally Chivers suggested this interpretation to me.

17. Linda's judgmental attitude toward Maggie for being sexually promiscuous and her hierarchical description of orgasm as being "inferior" to her own pleasures are troubling; however, they are a powerful way of affirming her own asexual life at an immediate level. Furthermore, the film ends with some hope that Linda and Maggie can coexist with difference. It is important that the hierarchy between asexuality and sexuality has to be challenged in both ways.

18. Janice M. Irvine, "Regulated Passions: The Invention of Inhibited Sexual Desire and Sexual Addiction," in *Deviant Bodies: Critical Perspectives on Difference in Science and Popular Culture*, ed. Jennifer Terry and Jacqueline Urla (Bloomington: Indiana University Press, 1995), 327.

13

Be Prepared

S. LOCHLANN JAIN

I don't blame people for not knowing how to engage with a person with cancer. How would they? Heck, I hadn't either. Despite the fact that each year 70,000 Americans between the ages of fifteen and forty are diagnosed with the disease and that incidence in this age group has doubled in the last thirty years, many of my friends in their thirties have never had to deal with it on a personal level.

I remember when my cousin Elise was undergoing chemotherapy treatment while in her early thirties. When I met her I couldn't even mention it, couldn't (or wouldn't, or didn't) say that I was sorry or ask her how it was going—even though it was so obviously the thing that was going on. I was thirty-five for God's sake, a grown-up, a professional, a parent, and cancer was so unthinkable that I couldn't even acknowledge her disease. When my former partner's sister showed up at our house all bald after her chemotherapy, my only remark was, "Hey, you could totally be a lesbian." I was terrified, or in denial. More likely I had picked up the culture of stigma and this disabled me from giving genuine acknowledgment. But whatever sympathetic spin you want to put on it, I sucked in all the ways that I had to learn how to deal with later. Indeed, an assumption of exceptionalism was only the flip side of my own shame.

Fantasies of agency steep both sides of diagnosis. On the "previvor" side, images continually tell us that cancer can be avoided if you eat right, avoid Teflon and smoking, and come from strong stock. Alternatively, tropes of hope, survivorship, battling, and positive attitude are fed to people post-diagnosis as if they were at the helm of a ship in known waters, not along stormy and uncharted shores. And yet, so little of cancer science, patient experience, or survival statistics seems to provide backing for the ubiquitous calls for hope in the popular culture of cancer. After all, who would celebrate a survivor who did not stand amid at least a few poor SOBs who fell?

Everyone who has "battled," "been touched by," "survived," been "made into a shadow of a former self," or has been called to inhabit the myriad cancer clichés has been asked to live in a caricature. As poets say in rendering their craft, clichés serve to shut down meaning. Clichés allow us not to think about what we are describing or hearing about: we know roses are red. People with cancer are called to live in and through—even if recalcitrantly—these hegemonic clichés by news articles, TV shows, detection campaigns, patient pamphlets, high-tech protocol-driven treatments, hospital organizations and smells, and everyday social interactions. Such cultural venues as marches for hope, research funding and direction, pharmaceutical interests, survivor rhetoric, and hospital ads constitute not distinct cultural phenomena, but overlap to form a broader hegemony of ways that cancer is talked about and that in turn control and diminish the ways that cancer culture can be inhabited and spoken about. Cancer exceeds the biology of multiplying cells. But the paradoxes of cancer culture can also be used to reflect on broader American understandings of health and the mismatch of normative assumptions with the ways people actually live and die. The restricted languages of cancer are not innocent.

For an example of how individuated agency is used in cancer, one might look to the massive literature and movement spurred by Bernard Siegel, which is based in the moral complex of cancer and what he describes as the "exceptional patient." In *Love, Medicine, and Miracles: Lessons Learned about Self-Healing from a Surgeon's Experience with Exceptional Patients*, Siegel writes about having the right attitude to survive cancer.[1] In Siegel's view and its variants, surviving cancer becomes a moral calling, as if dying indicates some personal failure. Siegel-style literature offers another form of torture to people with cancer: Did my mind declare war on my body? Am I a cold, repressed person? (Okay, don't answer that.) This huge and punishing industry preys on fear as much as any in the cancer complex and adds guilt to the mix. As one woman with metastatic colon cancer said on a retreat I attended, "Maybe I haven't laughed enough. But then I looked around the room and some of you laugh a lot more than I do and you're still here." She died a year later, though she laughed plenty at the retreat.

It's no wonder that shame is such a common response to diagnosis. The dictionary helps with a description of shame: "The painful emotion arising from the consciousness of something dishonoring, ridiculous, or indecorous in one's own conduct or circumstances, or of being in a situation which offends one's sense of modesty or decency."[2] Indeed, cancer does offend. People in treatment are often advised to wear wigs and other disguises, to joke with colleagues; they are given tips on how to make others feel more at ease. One does want to present decency, to seem upbeat. And so do others. A quick "you look good," with a response of "oh, thanks," offers a welcome segue to the next discussion topic and enables a certain propriety to circumscribe the confusion of proper responses to illness, to the stigma embodied by the possibility of a short life and a painful death. One person with metastatic disease calls herself, semi-facetiously, "everyone's worst nightmare." Others speak about how hard it is to see the celebration of survivors while knowing that they themselves are being killed by the disease.

Social grace is a good thing. But given the scope of the disease—half of all Americans die of it and many more go through treatment—one might wonder what or whom such an astonishing cultural oversight serves. After all, how can cancer, a predictable result of an environment drowning in industrial and military toxicity, be dishonoring or indecorous? I don't mean its side effects; the physical breakdown of the body is perhaps definitive of the word "indecorous." But these pre- and post-diagnosis calls to disavowal can help illuminate the ugly underside of American's constant will to health, its normative assumptions about health and the social, individual, and generational traumas that it propagates. Expectations and assumptions about life span and their discriminatory and generational effects offer but one of many venues for such an exploration.

Survivorship in America

Perhaps it's a class issue, but I didn't really think about survival until I was called to consider being in the position of the one who might *be* survived. I was just tootling along until I was invited by diagnosis to inhabit this category, to attend retreats, camps, and support groups, to share an infusion room—to do all kinds of things with many people who have not, in fact, survived cancer—and thus to survive them at their memorial services, the garage sales of their things, and in the constructing and reading of memorial Websites and obituaries.

To be sure, cancer survivorship (as opposed to either cancer death or just plain survival) comes with its benefits. I got a free kayak, albeit with a leak. When things are going really wrong I think about how my life insurance could pay for some cool things for my kids, or that maybe I don't have to worry about saving for a down payment since in order for a home to be a good investment you should really plan to live in it for five years. Sometimes, when you find yourself buying into those cancer mantras of living in the moment, you can look around from a superior place at all the people scurrying around on projects you have determined do not matter—and then go and do the laundry or shop for groceries, just like everyone else. Or like Bette Davis does in the movie *Dark Victory* as she dies of a brain tumor, you can consider yourself the lucky one, not having to survive the deaths of those you love. You have that strange privilege of being able to hold the materiality of your own mortality up against every attempt to make value stick. You may wonder, as I do, how anyone survives the death of a parent or a sibling or a close friend or lover—the things that are purportedly normal life events— until you go through it yourself.[3]

On the other hand, it may be easy to devolve into the narcissism of unremitting fear. I like to keep in mind what a driver once told me when I asked him what it was like to drive celebrities such as Oprah Winfrey around New York. He said, "They like to think they are important. But after every funeral I've been to, people do the saaaaame thing. They eat."

The doctor survives the clinical trial, the child survives the parent, the well survive the sick. But how have we come to take this survivorship for granted, as something to which we are entitled? Even a century or two ago there would have been a good chance that several of us would have died in childbirth or of some illness. Devastating as it may have been, we would have expected this. And we don't exactly live in a medical nirvana. The United States is not even in the top ten for the longevity of its population. In fact, the United States is missing from the top twenty or even thirty for longevity in the world. In some studies, it's not even in the top forty.[4] Despite this statistic, the United States spends more than any other nation on health care. Part of Americans' dismal life expectancy results from the broad lack of access to health care as well as the broader and well-documented discrimination in health care against the usual suspects: African Americans, women, younger people, and queers. But other factors that affect even those with excellent access to excellent care play in as well: the high levels of toxins in the environment, including those in human and animal bodies; cigarettes; guns; little oversight for food, automobile, and other product safety; high rates of medical error.

In short, despite the insistent rhetoric of health, American economies simply do not prioritize it. That's okay. There is no particular reason that the general health of a population should trump all other concerns. But given the evidence, how do we come to believe this disconnect between dismal health status in the United States and the entitlement to normative health and life span? What kind of management has this necessary disavowal required? And what about the obverse of this question: how do these stories constitute those who are forced to drop out? After all, if survival is a moral and financial

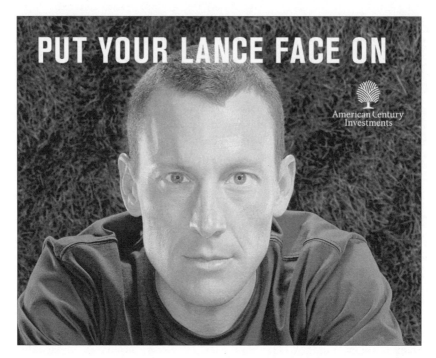

Figure 13.1: The 2006 "Put Your Lance Face On" campaign from American Century Investments. This version of the promotional photo omits the warning, required in print advertisement publications, that it is possible to lose money by investing (included in the original).

expectation and entitlement, then mortality must be constituted as something outside of normal life, even though these early deaths pay for pensions and other deferred payments. Even though everyone will die. I hypothesize that stigma and shame offer a way to examine and challenge ideals of health and the ways that normative life spans have been constructed.

Accumulation

For analytical wealth in this matter, nothing beats a recent advertisement for American Century Investments that featured Lance Armstrong (figure 13.1).

Armstrong has provided something of a translational figure for the nexus of industry, cancer, and humanitarianism that constitutes the discourses of cancer survivorship, foregrounding and even heroizing cancer survivors. His own story relentlessly underpins this cultural work.

While some accounts of Armstrong's success go so far as to credit chemotherapy for literally rebuilding his body as a cycling machine, and others link his drive and success to his cancer experience, Armstrong continually presents himself in public as a survivor, claiming that his greatest success and pride is having survived cancer. In his autobiography, *It's Not About the Bike*, Armstrong describes how, when diagnosed with testicular cancer in 1996, he actively sought the best care available to overcome a poor prognosis. He chose a doctor who offered a then-new treatment that turned out to revolutionize the treatment for testicular cancer, turning the disease from a high-risk cancer to a largely curable one even in its metastatic iteration. This coincidence in the timing of his disease and this new treatment has enabled him to make his own agency in finding medical care into another inspirational aspect of his cancer survival story.

In fact, cancer treatments are some of the most rote, protocol-driven treatments in medical practice, perfect examples of what historian Charles Rosenberg has detected as the rationalization of disease and diagnosis at the expense of the humanness of individual patients.[5] Yet Armstrong's story serves several purposes. It overemphasizes the role of agency in the success of cancer treatment, a view that correlates well with the advertising messages of high-profile cancer centers. It overestimates the curative potential of treatments for most cancers, something we would all like to believe in. And it propagates the myth that everyone has the potential to be a survivor—even as, ironically, survivorship against the odds requires the deaths of others.

This Armstrong story comes with real social costs for many people surviving with and dying of cancer. Miriam Engelberg's graphic novel, like so many cancer narratives, ends abruptly with the recurrence of her metastatic disease and her subsequent death. One prominent page of her book has a cartoon with her holding a placard stating, "Lance had a different cancer," in response to her friends' and colleagues' comparison of her with Armstrong and their terrifying denial of her actual situation.[6] So, while many cancer survivors consider Armstrong an icon and inspiration, others feel that he is misrepresentative of the disease. He at once gives them impossible standards of survivorship while at the same time building his heroism on the high death rates of other cancers.

The American Century Investments advertisement summons the reader to "Put Your Lance Face On." After gazing into the close-up image of a determined looking Armstrong and thinking quietly to oneself, "what the fuck?" one reads that "putting on a Lance face" "means taking responsibility for your future. . . . It means staying focused and determined in the face of challenges. When it comes to investing . . ." This ad is about Lance the Cyclist, sure; it is also about Lance the Cancer Survivor. Control over one's future holds together the common thread of cancer survival, Tour de France victory, and smart investing. But all this folds into the tiny hedge at the bottom of the ad: "Past performance is no guarantee of future results . . . it is possible to lose money by investing." Even the Lance Face can see only so far into the future.

This warning, necessary by law, echoes a skill essential to living in capitalism. In her study of market traders, Caitlyn Zaloom finds that "a trader must learn to manage both his own engagements with risk and the physical sensations and social stakes that accompany the highs and lows of winning and losing. . . . Aggressive risk taking is established and sustained by routinization and bureaucracy; it is not an escape from it."[7] The conflation of Armstrong as athlete and cancer survivor in this ad offers the perfect personification of market investing, since the healthy functioning of a capitalist order requires a valorization of focused determination and responsibility for one's future. By now a truism, liberal economic and political ideals require citizens to place themselves within a particular masochistic relationship to time. What else but an ethos of deferred gratification would allow such retirement plans to remain solvent?

As offensive as this ad is in its use of disease to create business, Armstrong's story constitutes a culturally acceptable version of courage, cancer, and survival that serves to comfort a population with increasing cancer rates, and the ad puts to use and propagates these notions of survivorship. As one person wrote about giving Armstrong's autobiography to her mother as she was dying of cancer, "I wanted her to be a courageous 'survivor' too. I think we find it less creepy or at least difficult when people assume the role of survivor, where they pretend they're going to live an easy and long life."[8]

You can be angry at cancer; you can battle cancer. One campaign underwritten by a company that builds radiation technology even allows people to write letters to cancer. But to be angry at the culture that produces the disease and disavows it as a horrible death is to be a poor sport, to not live up to the expectations of the good battle and the good death witnessed everywhere in cancer obituaries. A bad attitude of this genre certainly will never enable you to become an exceptional patient. It's as though a death threat blackmails cancer anger and frustration. But more astonishing still is the way in which this "poor sport" characterization carries over even into other cancer events.

There is nothing wrong with having fun while making money. As one under-forty person who has been living in the cancer complex for over two decades said, "A fundraiser is where you invite people to a big fun event, serve great drinks, and do everything possible for them *not* to think about cancer."[9] You do want people to feel good and strong so that they will open their wallets, but this humanitarian charity model ("Swim for women with cancer!") obscures the politics and paradoxes of such divisions. As one person organizing a fundraiser for her particular and rare cancer said as she thought about asking her doctors to attend her event, "They've made enough money off my cancer, they could pay some back."[10] I signed on as the mixologist for the event and spent several hours designing circus-themed drinks with little cotton candy garnishes.

Time and Accumulation

Armstrong's class, gender, and curable cancer allow his iconic status to overshadow the simple fact that cancer can completely destroy your financial savings and your family's future. Sixty percent of personal bankruptcies in the United States result from the high cost of health care.[11] This news, wonderful for people working in the healthcare industry since many people will pay anything for medical goods and services, means that cancer can be a long, expensive disease, paid for over generations.

When one's financial planner asks, semi-ironically, how long you plan to live, he calls up the paradox of survivorship. Middle- and upper-class Americans are asked to plan for an assumed longevity, and to be sure, a properly planned life span combined with a little luck comes with its rewards. But in times of trouble, the language of financial service starts to show cracks, even for healthy youngish people. The other day, when interviewing a Fidelity representative about my decreasing retirement account, the representative kept using the phrase "as your retirement plan grows." When I pointed out that it had, in fact, shrunk by 45 percent, he just stared at me blankly. When, as an experiment, I asked him about people who don't make it to the age of sixty-five, he pleaded, "You really need to think about it as a retirement plan."

No matter how we are interpellated to think about these accounts, non-normative life spans tell us about the ways that capitalist notions of time and accumulation work both economically and culturally. Many kinds of economic benefits, for example, are based in an implied life span: you work now, and we'll pay you later. Social Security benefits are granted on the basis of how much you have put into the system over the years, and they last until you or your survivors are no longer eligible. Middle-class jobs often include not only salaries, but what are known as "deferred payments." Pensions fall into this category, as do penalty-free retirement savings, and the benefit some academics get of partial payment of their children's tuition.

If you croak, some of these contributions may revert back to your estate; others may be disbursed to qualifying survivors; others will be recycled into the plans that will pay for the education of your colleagues' children. As with any insurance policy, such calculations require that the state or the employer offer salary packages in the form of a financial hedge on your mortality and calculate the averages over the whole workforce. Payments for those who get old depend on the fact that some will die young. It's not personal; it's statistical.

Actually, I take that back. I guess there is not much that is more personal than your sex life, and if you are heterosexual and married—that is, if you say you are sleeping with one person only and that person is of the opposite sex and over a certain age—your cancer card will play more lucratively. If you fit these criteria, you may be able to pass on these benefits and enable your loved ones to pay off some of your medical debts or provide a way toward a more comfortable life in (and sometimes because of) your absence. The survivorship of a spouse is a state-endowed right, enabled in the form of a cash benefit and various forms of tax relief. A husband's or wife's death will enable his or her spouse to receive Social Security checks for decades. This cash enables a sort of proxy-survival by fulfilling your responsibility toward the support of your spouse and possibly the support of your children.

This is precisely how one person explained to me his reasoning behind a recent change of genders: he can now legally have a wife, legally bring her into the country, and legally offer her the protections of Social Security. For the same reasons, my lawyer advised me to marry a man, so that my husband could give the survivor-cash to my girlfriend. For the same reasons, my mother was bummed out when I turned out not to be straight. Health is social and institutional as well as physical. Capital and family legitimate and live through each other, in some sense rendering each other immortal.[12]

Social Security might be seen as ensuring that those who do not conform to its measures of social legitimacy—people with forms of support that do not fall into the marriage category—are not given the forms of security into which they are asked to pay while they live. Straight marriage presents a form of cultural longevity for the institution of marriage, and the labor of those who cannot partake in such survivorship literally underwrites the security of the individuals who can.[13]

Historians of marriage have documented how ideas about the well-being of children led to these forms of social support. But take a closer look, and you will see that it's only some children who benefit from these protective policies. Here's an example. My employer offers a housing benefit that gives some employees financial assistance in purchasing a house. It also describes death as a "severed relationship." The relationship between my employer and an employee of the university can pass through a surviving partner—they included same-sex couples in their benefits plan in 1992, albeit as taxable benefits rather than the untaxed benefits that straight people receive—such that a surviving partner may continue to live in a house purchased with the help of this fringe benefit. However, if an employee has children and no partner, the relationship is severed and the children are "SOL" (shit out of luck); they must sell the house no matter what the market is like and return the down payment loan to the employer. The debt cycles of illness and the early deaths of a parent are thus differently borne out through what counts as legitimate survival, thus reinforcing and rewarding normative social structures.

But more important to my argument here, these retirement and Social Security benefits offer one means by which the terms of life span come to be taken for granted by the middle class in the United States. They make life span into a financial and moral calling, albeit one that the state will be willing to partially subsidize in the event of the deaths of the citizens who fulfill its principles of economic and sexual responsibility.

All this rests on a premise critical to economies in America: time and accumulation go together. You need the former to get the latter, and you have more stuff as you get older. No wonder people want to freeze themselves. Seriously. Cryonics offers an obvious strategy to maximize capitalist accumulation. On my salary, I'll be able to pay for my kids' college tuition in one hundred and fifty years. If I could freeze myself and my daughters and let my savings grow over that time, then come back to life after all the work of accumulation has been done for me, well, I could take full advantage of both the deferral and the gratification.[14] This may sound ludicrous, but it's basically the next step of what is already happening; people already freeze their eggs and sperm in order to maintain their fertility to a point at which they have gained the sort of financial security that time and accumulation (are supposed to) bring.

While cryonics suspends biological life as capitalism proliferates, uncontrollably duplicating cells work to immobilize biological life. Cancer parodies excess. It could not be farther from the metaphors of an external enemy attacking the body imagined by visions of targeted chemotherapy, the broad political imaginary of the war on cancer, or the trope of the courageously battling and graciously accepting patient. If wealth rots the soul, accumulating tumors rot the host. It just grows, sometimes as a tumor you should have noticed but didn't, sometimes as a tumor you can't help but notice but can't remove. It may just live there; you may touch it each day. It may disappear or it may wrap its way around your tongue. Either way, its changing size may make it seem living or dying. It inhabits a competing version of time, not yours, to which such things as savings and retirement are supposed to correlate, but its own, to which such words as "apoptosis" and "runaway" accrue. These versions of competing time reveal a lot about life spans in capitalism.

Conclusion

Alas, the Lance Face aims not toward the growing demographic of cancer survivors whose bodies experience the fissures of the immortal pretensions of economic time. Unlike many people who calculate their odds and cash out their retirement policies after diagnosis, or the friends of mine who told me that I was the inspiration for them to live in the moment and renovate their home, or those ads that regularly appear in *Cure* magazine that offer to buy the life insurance policies of people with cancer in exchange for a percentage, the Lance ad replays tiresome injunctions to future thinking, saving, and determination. The ad encourages the potential consumer of banking products to work in the broader interests of capital. Simply put, the ad uses cancer for its own ends and is able to do so because of the way that cancer rhetorics have so unquestioningly overlapped with notions of progress and accumulation in capitalism.

The cultural management of cancer terror follows to some extent the Cold War strategies of damping nuclear terror. You may have wondered why the phrase "you are the bomb" presents itself as something of a compliment whereas, in a romantic situation, the comment "you are the gas chamber" may not go over that well. Anthropologist Joseph Masco has analyzed how Americans didn't just turn the threat of nuclear annihilation into atomic cafes, bikinis, and B-52 cocktails on their own; we were taught to survive through specific governmental programs sought to manage the emotional politics of the bomb. Nuclear terror, as a paralyzing emotion, was converted into nuclear fear, "an affective state that would allow citizens to function in a time of crisis."[15] Such emotional management required a two-pronged approach. First, citizens were asked to "take responsibility for their own survival." Second, enemy status was displaced from nuclear war onto public panic, such that the main threat was perceived as inappropriate reactions to detonation, rather than to the bomb itself. Even with increased bomb testing and its release of radiation into the atmosphere, the discovery of high levels of radiation in American flesh and teeth, and the corresponding increasing of cancer rates along fallout routes and among nuclear workers, the nuclear threat was always constituted as coming from the outside, never as the predictable and calculated risk of American nuclear programs. In that sense, the forms of emotional management that resulted from military technologies underpin cancer culture in the United States as much as the technologies of chemotherapy and radiation do.

To be sure, the increasing use of the language of survivorship in mainstream cancer culture offers a welcome change from the days when people with cancer were asked to use plastic cutlery so as not to infect those around them or were not told of their diagnoses in order to protect them. Now, the person who survives cancer walks a fine line between courage and deception, horror and the quotidian, in ensuring that American models of health retain their normative status. Lance Armstrong offers the perfect venue for such disavowals, as he currently rises as if in a second coming, high above the Nike building at Union Square in San Francisco and other American cities, his Lance face in perfect shape, with another sufficiently vague, sportsmanly tag line: "Hope Rides Again."

What if, instead of some broad and grammatically, if not affectively, meaningless aim as marching and riding "for hope," fundraisers attempted to ban any one of the thousands of known carcinogens in legal use? What if we walked, ran, swam, rode not for hope, but against PAH, MTBE, BPA or any other common carcinogen? Such an effort would require naming the problem rather than the symptom, and recognizing how we are all implicated. It would require that we invest in cancer culture not as a node of sentimentality but as a basic fact of American life.

NOTES

1. Bernie S. Siegel, *Love, Medicine, and Miracles: Lessons Learned about Self-Healing from a Surgeon's Experience with Exceptional Patients* (New York: Harper and Row, 1986).

2. *Oxford English Dictionary*, 2nd ed., s.v. "Shame."

3. Again, I think it is easier to speak facetiously from the position of having a non-metastatic diagnosis.

4. Stephen Ohlemachter, "US Slipping in Life Expectancy Rankings," *Washington Post*, August 12, 2007, http://www.washingtonpost.com/wp-dyn/content/article/2007/08/12/AR2007081200113.html.

5. See Charles E. Rosenberg, "The Tyranny of Diagnosis: Specific Entities and Individual Experience," *The Milbank Quarterly* 80, no. 2 (June 2002): 237–60.

6. Miriam Engelberg, *Cancer Made Me a Shallower Person* (New York: Harper, 2006).

7. Caitlin Zaloom, "The Productive Life of Risk," *Cultural Anthropology* 19, no. 3 (August 2004): 365.

8. Personal correspondence with author, April 10, 2008.

9. Personal correspondence with author, March 15, 2009.

10. Personal correspondence with author, April 11, 2009.

11. See David U. Himmelstein, Deborah Thorne, Elizabeth Warren, and Steffie Wool-handler, "Medical Bankruptcy in the United States, 2007: Results of a National Study," *The American Journal of Medicine* 122, no. 8 (August 2009): 741–46.

12. These structures carry invisible costs even for straight people who believe themselves to be outside of these cycles. Think for example of the shooting of Harvey Milk and George Moscone. The short sentence given to Dan White for the shooting is usually ascribed to the fact that, since Milk was queer, the judge believed that his life was not worth much. Moscone was considered collateral damage. See *The Times of Harvey Milk*, dir. Rob Epstein, 90 min., Black Sand Productions, 1984.

13. This kind of structural attention to cultural institutions and actual care are understudied. For example, when President Barack Obama made an exception to his usual homophobic platform to call for allowing same-sex couples to be able to visit their partners in hospitals, he was making a way for partners to be able to love each other and to be able to share a deep experience. Advocacy and protection are huge parts of contemporary medical care. I have come across hundreds of examples of this in my years of research. This aspect of contemporary medical care includes everything from making sure that medical records are transferred properly or read, that medical allergies are made known, that machinery is working, that people wash their hands and are given the proper doses of medication. Such bedside advocacy is an enormous, and understudied, part of healthcare provision.

14. Tiffany Romain is working on an important dissertation on this subject in the Department of Anthropology at Stanford University.

15. Joseph Masco, "Survival Is Your Business: Engineering Ruins and Affect in Nuclear America," *Cultural Anthropology* 23, no. 2 (May 2008): 366.

14

In the Name of Pain

TOBIN SIEBERS

To be against health is to be for pain because human beings suffer from sickness. But to suffer from sickness is something of a metaphor. We supposedly *suffer* from diseases and disabilities whether or not they are painful. The man standing on the corner pointing the white cane suffers from blindness, but he has no pain in his eyes or anywhere else. The young woman walking to the local deaf club suffers from deafness, but her body does not hurt and she seems perfectly happy. The Iraq war veteran suffers from quadriplegia, although he cannot feel a thing in most of his body.

A disabled body is supposedly a body in pain, and pain represents for most people a source of terror and an affront to human dignity. Nothing seems more horrifying to human beings than to imagine a lifetime of future suffering. Pain is, however, notoriously subjective. The usual observation notes that it is difficult to share pain, that one person cannot really understand the pain of another.[1] But a second difficulty exists—quite the opposite—and it is rarely discussed: how frequently people impute feelings of pain and suffering to other people. It is astonishing how often one person assumes that another person is in pain based solely on appearance or circumstances. Passersby approach the man standing on the corner with the white cane and gush with great admiration over his bravery in the face of suffering and adversity. They blurt out to the young deaf woman that they themselves could not bear such hardship. Complete strangers feel compelled to tell the paralyzed veteran that they would rather be dead than be him. Such reactions may set off feelings of grief in the objects of pity if they are genuinely in pain, but they may just as likely respond with bewilderment to the fact that their happy existence represents a lifetime of suffering to absolute strangers who know nothing about their families, occupations, physical conditions, or daily circumstances. Such is the nature of pain in the human universe. In an instant and with little reflection, pain triggers powerful emotions, opinions, and judgments.

To speak in the name of pain is to resist these bad habits of thought. Pain is a motive force rarely questioned and stunning in its ability to engage us in or disengage us from the lives of other human beings. It raises money for charities. It drives legislation. It starts and ends wars. It justifies the ending of life and the refusal to begin it. It is at the heart of debates about abortion, assisted suicide, wrongful birth, neonatal testing, end-of-life care, right to life, and mercy killing. The philosophical school of utilitarianism judges life invalid by the quantity of its suffering, but utilitarianism has no premium on the distaste for pain and its use as a measure to make moral judgments.[2] On the subject of pain, there are few non-utilitarians.

What does it mean to speak in the name of pain in such a world? For one thing, it is to court the accusation of masochism. There are those who take pleasure in pain, and some disabled people find in masochism a way to manage their disabilities. For instance, Bob Flanagan, a "super masochist," had cystic fibrosis, a condition that often proves fatal at an early age. His engagement with masochism allowed him psychological and physical control over his body, presumably contributing to his long life span.[3] He died at age forty-three, one of the oldest survivors of the disease. Flanagan's choice is not for everyone, but it does suggest that pain has a more complicated relation to quality of life than most people wish to admit. It is crucial, then, to understand that pain may sometimes actively improve quality of life.

My claim here is not made in the name of masochism. Rather, I speak in the name of pain to reveal that the fear of pain is one of the most pervasive and insidious justifications of disability oppression.[4] Disabled people are stigmatized almost everywhere, carved up by doctors in unnecessary surgeries, and often lose their lives because other people wrongly assume that they are in pain. Furthermore, disabled people who are actually in pain are subjected to the same horrific treatment because they can mount no argument justifying a life in any way thought by others to be painful. Pain is a motive force impossible at the present moment to contradict. A painful life is simply considered a life not worth living. A painful life is easily terminated without objection. A painful life is not thought to be a *human* life, and people with disabilities can be tortured and killed in the name of whatever pain's opposite is—certainly not pleasure, but a panoply of concepts that questions the value of any life possessing even the most meager association with pain.

The use of pain as a motive force to justify disability oppression is most visible in events that make the headlines. No one knows what harm the fear of pain causes in the more quiet and secluded realm of private life, in the everyday occurrences that do not catch wind in the media but remain hidden in small family dramas. The damage must be enormous. Headline events are fewer but knowable. They are global, testifying to the fact that pain holds sway over moral and political judgment irrespective of cultural belief. They are also controversial, fortunately, and this sometimes creates an opportunity to think about both sides of the question of pain, opposing those who think that pain must always be the deciding factor in quality of life to those rare individuals who take a different point of view.

Recently in the United States, a firestorm of controversy arose around the case of Seattle's Ashley X, sometimes called the "Pillow Angel." Ashley was born with cerebral palsy; she cannot hold up her head, change the position of her body, walk, or talk. She is understood to be profoundly cognitively disabled.[5] But her parents say that she is alert and loves music, that she seems to watch television, vocalizes in response to music and attention, and goes to school. Nevertheless, her parents induced a medical state of permanent pre-pubescence in their daughter at the age of six by surgically removing her breast buds and uterus and by placing her on a high dose of estrogen to stunt her growth. They also had her appendix removed. Their goal is to keep Ashley as small as possible, making it easier both to control her and to move her from place to place. "We call her our 'Pillow Angel,'" her parents explain, "since she is so sweet and stays right where we place her—usually on a pillow."[6]

At the heart of the controversy is the question of whether Ashley's parents are rescuing their daughter from pain or abusing her, but pain remains in either case the deciding factor. When in 2006, the parents went public with the "Ashley Treatment," they found themselves in the middle of a national controversy about the injury of disabled people. Involuntary sterilization and unnecessary surgeries for the convenience of institutions (such as the removal of teeth) have long been discarded as barbaric, but the Seattle Children's Hospital carried out the Ashley Treatment anyway, admitting three years later that its actions were illegal. Activists in the disability community attacked Ashley's parents for violating her human rights and abusing her, and demanded a condemnation of her doctors by the American Medical Association, but no response was forthcoming from either legal or medical authorities. Ashley's parents continue to defend their actions in the name of reducing their daughter's pain, and many people accept their motives because they too fear pain above all else and consequently identify with the desire to rescue the young woman from imagined future suffering. Her parents claim that they are saving Ashley from the pain of menstrual cramps, that having large breasts is "uncomfortable," "could sexualize" her and invite "abuse," that having an appendix places her at a 5 percent risk of appendicitis, that her low body weight protects her against "bed sores," "pneumonia," and "bladder infections," and that the hysterectomy eliminates "the possibility of uterine cancer and other common and often painful complications" affecting women later in life.[7] Ashley's parents explicitly connect the avoidance of pain and suffering to their daughter's quality of life and state with confidence that God is on their side: "The God we know wants Ashley to have a good quality of life. . . . Knowingly allowing avoidable suffering for a helpless and disabled child can't be a good thing in the eyes of God."[8] To my knowledge, only one commentator questions the sincerity of Ashley's parents on the issue of pain. Patricia Williams asks why, if the avoidance of pain is the deciding factor, Ashley's parents stopped short of performing other invasive medical procedures to protect their daughter against suffering: "Why not remove all her teeth to spare her the pain of cavities? Why not excise her fingernails to spare her the pain of accidentally scratching herself?"[9] Unfortunately, if Ashley's parents had resorted to these procedures, few people would have questioned their motives, so profound is the prejudice against pain.

A painful life is a wrongful life. Not many people seem to disagree with this proposition. Indeed, the idea of a wrongful life lies behind practices that range from those depriving disabled people of their civil and human rights to those justifying their deaths. In France, the idea of wrongful life made headlines when the parents of Nicolas Perruche brought suit against a doctor and medical laboratory for making mistakes that resulted in his mother choosing to give birth rather than to abort him. Josette Perruche discovered early in her pregnancy that her four-year-old daughter had contracted rubella. She asked her doctor to test her for the disease because it can produce severe disabilities in pregnancy, stating that she preferred to have an abortion if she was exposed. The doctor and laboratory responded incorrectly that the fetus was not infected. Nicolas Perruche was born profoundly incapacitated: deaf, almost blind, and with cognitive disabilities. The Perruches sued the doctors and laboratory for malpractice and won the suit. They eventually sued them again, this time demanding damages for causing him to be born and asking to be compensated for the lifetime cost of caring for their disabled child.

The Cour de Cassation, France's Supreme Court, ruled in favor of the plaintiffs, and although its decision never mentioned the concepts of "wrongful birth" or "wrongful life," the ruling was interpreted as protecting the right not to be born.[10] The judgment was reiterated a year later when the same court found that children with Down syndrome have the legal right never to have been born and can sue doctors for errors that resulted in their births. At the heart of wrongful life suits is the idea that plaintiff rights are violated by being born, that people have the right to be terminated before birth to avoid a life pronounced painful and miserable. In effect, the court's ruling confirms a belief in the concept of a "wrong life," that is, a life less worthy than others, a life without human dignity, a life not worth living. In the case of disabled people, it seems, death is preferable to life.

In a world where pain represents the ultimate measure of quality of life, all disabled people risk having their existences described as wrongful because disability and suffering are thought synonymous. Disabled lives are routinely described as lives not worth living, lives undeserving of human dignity, lives judged inferior to death. The "Affaire Perruche," as it came to be known in France, provoked an uproar over these ideas, questioning common perceptions about disability. The court appeared to suggest that being born with a disability is a wrong in itself, apparently because disability produces exceptional costs. Jean-François Mattéi, head of the conservative Liberal Democratic Party, attacked the decision before the National Assembly, claiming that the court seemed "to validate the principle that the birth of a disabled child would be in itself an anomaly."[11] Jerry Sainte-Rose, the French Advocate General, objected to the decision with precise reasoning. According to the court, he stated, "The wrong is the life, and the absence of the wrong is death." He warned that the ruling would lead to a "precautionary eugenics," introducing "discrimination between parents of good biological quality and other parents who should abstain from procreating." He also cautioned that the decision would transform abortion from a choice into an "obligation."[12] Christine Boutin, speaking for the conservative Alliance for the Right to Life, agreed that the court decision "confirms France's entry into institutional eugenics."[13] The disability community in France raised alarms against the decision as well. "The Perruche ruling reveals the total incapacity of our society to see disability as a richness, and its rejection of anything that is different," Jean-Christophe Parisot, President of the Collective of Disabled Democrats, explained: "We have to break out of this spiral which condemns abnormality, and calls human beings 'mistakes.'"[14]

In January 2002, the National Assembly passed legislation that made the Perruche ruling obsolete. The legislation outlaws awarding damages solely as a result of birth and specifies that people born with disabilities may seek redress for the negligent acts that either caused or aggravated their disability. The new law seems like a victory for the disability community, and perhaps it is, but the Cour de Cassation has subsequently made rulings that permit plaintiffs to sue for lifetime damages against doctors whose malpractice brings disabled children into the world.

In the current climate, it is difficult to take one side over the other because both sides rely on the conception of disability as suffering. The French government speaks in the name of disabled people and against their suffering, but it also protects doctors from damages and rising insurance costs. The Cour de Cassation stands against medical and governmental authorities, recognizing that malpractice may result in the birth of disabled children and holding doctors responsible for the lifetime care of these children rather than limiting damages on purely economic and political grounds. And yet the concept of wrongful life, necessary to awarding these lifetime damages, stigmatizes people with disabilities as living painful lives less valuable and dignified than those of nondisabled people.

A final case, which might be called the case of the century, returns us to the United States and to the tragic death of Terri Schiavo—"the longest public execution in American history," according to Nat Hentoff.[15] The young woman existed in a brain-injured state for fifteen years before she lost the right to stay alive against the claim that her life was an offense to human dignity and not worth living. At the time of her death, 80 percent of the U.S. population said of Schiavo that they would not "want to live like that."[16] In 1990, Schiavo had collapsed from an unknown cause. The collapse resulted in severe damage to her cerebral cortex, but the base of her brain was left untouched. For the next decade and a half she lived, under the care of her parents and husband, without higher brain functions, but breathing on her own, with no ventilator or other medical technology to keep her alive except for the feeding tube through which she received food and water. Her husband and parents came to a bitter disagreement about her continued survival. Her husband, who was the court-appointed guardian, filed suit to have her feeding tube removed, while her parents opposed any attempt to end her life artificially and prematurely, pleading to be given her guardianship. Her husband refused, claiming that his wife would prefer to die rather than live in such a painful and diminished state.

Once the conflict became public, the court cases deciding Schiavo's life and death became part of a media circus concerning rights to life and death, abortion, end-of-life care, and other causes not entirely her own. The attention surrounding Schiavo produced a vast and largely contradictory set of images about her life, capacities, and circumstances. But one element remained consistent. Those who wished for her death and those who opposed it wanted equally to avoid making her suffer, demonstrating both the association of pain with disability and how pain takes on contradictory guises to serve different ends. In Schiavo's case more than any other seen in this chapter, the disabled person's suffering was presented as an affront to human dignity. Those in favor of Schiavo's death described her existence as a mockery of human life, as a miserable existence robbed of dignity, while those who sought to protect her described the efforts to take her life as an attack on human dignity. An effort by the state of Florida to pass legislation to save her was ruled unconstitutional, and the Florida Circuit Court later ordered that her feeding tube be removed and that no attempts be made to provide her with water or food by mouth.[17] Terri Schiavo was deprived of food and water at noon on March 18, 2005 and died thirteen days later of renal failure caused by dehydration.

On one side of the controversy, people felt that Schiavo had to die to preserve her humanity and dignity. Anna Quindlen in *Newsweek* magazine opposed the publication of photographs showing Schiavo in her disabled state, writing that "she should have been remembered for what she was, not what's left of her." Quindlen claimed that the "cruelest thing" that we can do to people in Schiavo's condition "is to force them to live."[18] No one was forcing Schiavo to live, since she had stayed alive for fifteen years without life support, but Quindlen, like many other Americans, confused her feeding tube with a ventilator, stating incorrectly that Schiavo was being "kept alive by extraordinary measures." Ellen Goodman, a nationally syndicated columnist, denied that Schiavo should be called disabled because she was too incapacitated to merit the label: "To describe Terri Schiavo as handicapped degrades the very term."[19] According to these commentators and to the courts, Schiavo's disability robbed her of dignity and humanity. For them, she existed in a state of suffering without the ability to communicate her pain to others. Compassion, humanity, and human dignity dictated that she be put out of her misery.

On the other side of the controversy, media commentators made the case that Schiavo was not suffering and that putting her to death would be not only unjust but also painful. Because she was not on life support, ending her life was not a simple matter of turning off a machine or pulling a plug. Putting her to death required extraordinary measures. In the case of capital punishment, the courts determine the method of execution, usually choosing the least painful one, although it is not clear what a painless death sentence is. In this case too, an act of violence was necessary if Schiavo was to stop living, but the courts could not rely on the usual methods of execution because she was not guilty of a capital offense. The legal decision to remove her feeding tube awkwardly mimicked the typical end-of-life choice to remove a dying person from a ventilator, except that Schiavo was not being kept alive by her feeding tube, and she could not be expected to die within minutes as someone removed from a ventilator would. That it took thirteen days for Schiavo to die exposes the extremes to which the courts went in their quest to end her life.

The fear of pain justifies irrational and often heinous acts against disabled people. These acts cannot really be defended on logical grounds. They are understandable, however, given a generous interpretation of the very real fear of human suffering. But no such fears seem to have protected Schiavo. While those calling for her death pronounced pain the ultimate enemy of humanity, they decided to kill her in the most brutal and painful way to safeguard her human dignity. People from opposing political camps in the United States agree on very little, but they agreed in this case that Schiavo's death was horrific. Andrew McCarthy in the *National Review*, a conservative publication, called Schiavo's death a "cold-blooded murder."[20] For McCarthy, the deprivation of water and food amounts to torture, and he noted that Florida anti-torture law, aptly called "Abuse, Neglect, and Exploitation of Elderly Persons and Disabled Adults," should have stopped the cruelty against Schiavo and placed her husband and the judge of the Florida Circuit Court under arrest. Stuart Taylor, Jr., a liberal-leaning commentator, called Schiavo's death "state-sanctioned death by dehydration."[21] Nat Hentoff, a libertarian columnist writing in the liberal *Village Voice*, described graphically for an uncaring public the effects on individuals of death by dehydration: "Their skin cracks, their tongue cracks, their lips crack. They may have nosebleeds because of the drying of the mucous membranes, and heaving and vomiting might ensue because of the drying out of the stomach lining. They feel the pangs of hunger and thirst. . . . It is an extremely agonizing death."[22] No criminal in U.S. history, many critics observed, has ever been executed as inhumanely by starvation and dehydration. Schiavo's situation was different for one reason only. "It is Ms. Schiavo's disability," Harriet McBryde Johnson wrote, "that makes her killing different in the eyes of the Florida courts."[23]

The fear of pain is often the beginning of oppression. But pain can also be the beginning of compassion. The idea is not to dismiss compassion as if it were oppression but to think about the difference between them, a difference not easily and reliably established but one that needs to be attempted nevertheless. Oppression puts the life of one kind of person below that of another. It fits one person's life to another life by conceiving of that kind of person as pliable, manageable, and submissive, as an inferior life designed for service to another by that other. Compassion feels with the other person, granting this person's life value equal to all other lives. It places itself in service to another life on the other person's terms, assuming the commitment to help this person find a life worthy of a human being, that is, a life at the heart of and embraced by other human beings.

Not every disabled person is in pain, but all people in chronic pain are disabled, and they face enormous oppression produced by the fear of pain. To speak in the name of pain is to feel for and with those people whose lives risk above all others being seen as not worth living, as undignified, as not human. It is to admit people in pain into the company of human beings with the assurance that human life will not suffer but prosper as a result. Martin Heidegger philosophizes that human beings only recognize the essence of human existence by confronting their "radical finitude"—the ineluctable fact that fragility defines each and every human life.[24] Mustering technology to rescue ourselves from our vulnerability, he claims, only makes our existence as human beings more machine-like and less human. There is disability in the future of every human life, and as long as the conflict between life and pain stands unquestioned, pain will continue to produce fears about the future. Parents will turn to medical technologies such as the Ashley Treatment to rescue their disabled children from suffering, radically limiting the possibilities of their future lives in the process. Other parents, gripped by the fear of pain, will understand the lives of their disabled children as wrongful in themselves, wishing that they had never been born. Everyone will find new reasons to kill disabled people who are thought, like Terri Schiavo, to have no future because they live with pain.

NOTES

1. Elaine Scarry, who argues that pain destroys language, provides the classic discussion about the inexpressibility of pain. See *The Body in Pain: The Making and Unmaking of the World* (New York: Oxford University Press, 1985), 19–20. See also Tobin Siebers, *Disability Theory* (Ann Arbor: University of Michigan Press, 2008), 203.

2. Certainly not the only but the most famous anti-disability rights utilitarian philosopher is Peter Singer, who believes

> that a being is a human being . . . is not relevant to the wrongness of killing it; it is, rather, characteristics like rationality, autonomy and self-consciousness that make a difference. Defective infants lack these characteristics. Killing them, therefore, cannot be equated with killing normal human beings, or any other self-conscious beings. This conclusion is not limited to infants who, because of irreversible mental retardation will never be rational, self-conscious beings. . . . Some doctors closely connected with children suffering from severe spina bifida believe that the lives of some of these children are so miserable that it is wrong to resort to surgery to keep them alive. . . . If this is correct, utilitarian principles suggest that it is right to kill such children.

See his *Practical Ethics* (New York: Cambridge University Press, 1979), 131–33.

3. "I was *forced* to be in the medical world," Flanagan explained, "so I turned that into something I could have control over instead of something that was controlling me." See Bob Flanagan, Andrea Juno, and V. Vale, *Bob Flanagan: Super-Masochist* (New York: Juno Books, 2000), 11. See also Dawn Reynolds on disability and BDSM in "Disability and BDSM: Bob Flanagan and the Case for Sexual Rights," *Sexuality Research & Social Policy* 4, no. 1 (2007): 40–52.

4. While it is important to distinguish empirically between physical and mental suffering, my analysis will focus on the refusal to make this distinction, a refusal characteristic of disability oppression. Disabled people manifest as suffering bodies, whether their pain is physical or mental and whether or not they are in pain. That the disabled body is represented as a suffering body, whatever the status of its pain, is a strong indication that disability oppression is at work. For an argument from the side of the medical model on the necessity of keeping separate pain and suffering, see Eric J. Cassell, *The Nature of Suffering and the Goals of Medicine* (New York: Oxford University Press, 1991).

5. On this issue, it is worth keeping in mind the story of Annie McDonald. McDonald was institutionalized at age three, supposed by her doctors and family to be profoundly cognitively disabled. At age sixteen she was offered a means of communication and she demonstrated that her cerebral palsy had not affected her intellect. Her story has many parallels with that of Ashley X. See her article, "The Other Story from a 'Pillow Angel': Been There. Done That. Preferred to Grow," *Seattle Post-Intelligencer*, June 18, 2007, http://seattlepi.nwsource.com/opinion/319702_noangel17.html.

6. "The 'Ashley Treatment,'" *Ashley Treatment*, posted January 2, 2007, http://ashleytreatment.spaces.live.com/.

7. The "Ashley Treatment" has emboldened other parents to take drastic actions to rescue their disabled children from future pain. In the United Kingdom, for example, Alison Thorpe asked surgeons at St. John's Hospital in Chelmsford to perform a hysterectomy and appendectomy on her disabled teenage daughter. Katie Thorpe, age fifteen, was born with cerebral palsy and has supposedly the intellectual ability of an eighteen-month-old child. Her mother argues that the surgery would take away the "pain and inconvenience of monthly periods," "the stomach cramps and the headaches, the mood swings, the tears." Medical authorities ruled against the mother's request on grounds that the procedures were medically unnecessary. See Sarah-Kate Templeton, "Disabled 15-Year-Old Girl to Lose Womb," *Sunday Times*, October 7, 2007, http://www.timesonline.co.uk/tol/news/uk/health/article2603965.ece. See also "Mother Seeks Girl's Womb Removal," *CNN.com*, October 12, 2007, http://edition.cnn.com/2007/HEALTH/10/08/hysterectomy/.

8. "The 'Ashley Treatment.'"

9. Patricia J. Williams, "Diary of a Mad Law Professor: Judge Not?" *The Nation*, March 12, 2007, http://www.thenation.com/doc/20070326/williams.
Other responses to the controversy focus on pain but predictably do not question its use as an agent of disability oppression. Peter Singer, who is on record as preferring death over disability, makes the typical utilitarian argument against suffering. He supports the "Ashley Treatment" and claims that "what matters in Ashley's life is that she should not suffer. . . . Lofty talk about human dignity should not stand in the way of children like her getting the treatment that is best both for them and their families." See his "A Convenient Truth," *New York Times*, January 26, 2007, http://www.nytimes.com/2007/01/26/opinion/26singer.html.

Speaking on behalf of the disability community, John Hockenberry disagrees with the treatment of Ashley. He argues that the role of any parent is to open their children to as many future opportunities as possible, concluding on this basis that Ashley's mother and father are no longer her parents because they treated her like "livestock" and made irrevocable decisions that have limited her future possibilities as much as her size. See his "Ashley X: Straight On Till Mourning," *The Blogenberry*, February 22, 2007, http://www.johnhockenberry.com/Blog/EDADA4E6-82AC-4B28-9525-3242F18F772A.html.

10. The legal distinction between "wrongful birth" and "wrongful life" comes down to whether disabled people may sue for simple medical damages or an entire lifetime of support based on the idea that every person possesses the right not to be born. For a clear discussion of the legal vocabulary and on the difference between wrongful life suits in France and the United States, see Therese M. Lysaught, "Wrongful Life? The Strange Case of Nicholas Perruche," *Commonweal* 129, no. 6 (March 22, 2002): 9–11, http://findarticles.com/p/articles/mi_m1252/is_6_129/ai_84817539.

11. As quoted in Acacio Pereria, "Un Handicapé né après une erreur médicale va être indemnisé," *Le Monde*, November 18–19, 2000, http://www.lemonde.fr/article/0,2320,seq-2079-118891-QUO,00.html.

12. As quoted in Elisabeth Fleury, "Né handicapé, Nicolas, 17 ans, sera indemnisé," Le Parisien, November 18, 2000.

13. Quoted in Pereria, "Un Handicapé."

14. As quoted in Hugh Schofield, "Disability Ruling Caused Huge Offence," *BBC News,* January 10, 2002, http://news.bbc.co.uk/2/hi/europe/1753065.stm.

15. Nat Hentoff, "Terri Schiavo: Judicial Murder," *Village Voice*, March 22, 2005, http://www.villagevoice.com/2005-03-22/news/terri-schiavo-judicial-murder/.

16. Ellen Goodman, "Schiavo's Lesson for Us All," *The Boston Globe*, March 31, 2005, http://www.boston.com/news/globe/editorial_opinion/oped/articles/2005/03/31/schiavos_lesson_for_us_all/.

17. Hentoff, "Terri Schiavo: Judicial Murder."

18. Anna Quindlen, "The Culture of Each Life," *Newsweek*, April 4, 2005, http://www.newsweek.com/id/49552.

19. Goodman, "Schiavo's Lesson for Us All."

20. Andrew McCarthy, "Is Prosecution the Solution?" *National Review*, March 20, 2005, http://www.nationalreview.com/mccarthy/mccarthy200503201334.asp.

21. Stuart Taylor, Jr., "What Terri Schiavo's Case Should Teach Us," *The Atlantic Monthly*, April 5, 2005, http://www.theatlantic.com/doc/200504u/nj_taylor_2005-04-05.

22. Hentoff, "Terry Schiavo: Judicial Murder." The autopsy on June 15, 2005 confirmed many facts about Schiavo's life and left others in dispute. It confirmed that Schiavo was not a terminal patient at the time when she was put to death, that she may have lived another ten years, and that healthcare officials administered morphine to her in the last days of life, even though her husband and his attorney had previously stated that she was in such a diminished state that she would not suffer during her termination. See Hentoff, "The Continuing Case of Terri Schiavo," *Jewish World Review*, July 11, 2005, http://www.jewishworldreview.com/cols/hentoff070705.asp. See also "Autopsy: No Sign Schiavo Was Abused," *CNN.com*, June 17, 2005, http://edition.cnn.com/2005/HEALTH/06/15/schiavo.autopsy/index.html.

The district medical examiner reported that she died of dehydration and that it was the most severe case he had ever seen. He also confirmed extensive damage to the cerebral cortex. See David Brown and Shailagh Murray, "Schiavo Autopsy Released," *Washington Post* (June 16, 2005), http://www.washingtonpost.com/wp-dyn/content/article/2005/06/15/AR2005061500512.html.

23. Harriet McBryde Johnson, "Not Dead At All: Why Congress Was Right to Stick Up for Terri Schiavo," *Slate*, March 23, 2005, http://www.slate.com/id/2115208/.

24. See Martin Heidegger, *Being and Time,* trans. John Macquarrie and Edward Robinson (New York: Harper, 1962).

15

Conclusion

What Next?

ANNA KIRKLAND

What should we do after deciding to be against health? What does it even mean to be against health? Should we stop going to the doctor or stop doing things that are supposed to be healthy? We do not conclude from the chapters collected here that it would be a good idea to start neglecting health. Rather, these chapters suggest an array of specific ways to be against certain formulations or political accounts of health. We propose a new recognition of the way health works socially, politically, emotionally, morally, globally, and personally that makes it impossible to invoke health in conventional ways. At the core of this proposal is the idea that the way one thinks about something like health really makes a difference in what it is and becomes. In other words, just seeing health from all the critical angles presented in this volume ought to mean that, even if we make the same health-related decisions as before, we nonetheless approach these decisions with new awareness. Of course, having read these chapters may mean making totally different health decisions, like not starting new diets or new medications.

The authors do more than just criticize health; they also offer alternative visions of what health could be. But first, what exactly are they against? Some critics hone in on the tedious moralism of health discourses. Richard Klein argues that scolding about health is not only unpleasant but can actually have iatrogenic or disease-producing effects. Kathleen LeBesco condemns fat hatred that is cloaked in health terms, and Joan Wolf points out how mean it is to harass bottle-feeding mothers with overstated health warnings. Eunjung Kim inverts the usual health/morality relationship, reminding us that now that regular sex is supposed to be health-enhancing, those who lead asexual lives find themselves stigmatized. One wrenching message to take away from Lochlann Jain's chapter is that on top of dealing with their disease, cancer patients are supposed to become virtuous survivors, "staying positive" to keep their cancer from returning. If it does, they not only face tough prognoses, but become blameworthy on more personal and moral terms.

Other critics are against the ways that talking about health obscures inequalities based on race and disability. Dorothy Roberts pushes back against race-based medicine, concerned that it participates too much in neoliberal demands that the individual fix herself and that it asks too little about why race-based health inequalities exist and persist. Tobin Siebers shares and amplifies Roberts's disability studies perspective, arguing that when we express concern about the pain someone else must surely be in, we are in part reacting to our own distaste for her disabled and devalued condition. Saying we want to prevent pain is similar to saying we want to promote health: it is so unassailable that we forget that there might be prejudice and irrational fear operating underneath those terms, keeping certain people in an unequal position.

For another set of critics in this book, the problem with the health/illness dichotomy is that it seems natural and real, but is actually created and marketed. Carl Elliott reminds us that the buying and selling of disease is a vast enterprise that relies on compelling claims to authority. A basic, cynical view of advertising in citizens' minds is not enough to compete with fake news produced by PR companies or manipulated studies funded by drug companies. At a time when we are being told more and more frequently to be personal stewards of our own health, the structural forces determining what information we have to make medical decisions are more and more complex, or at the very least, the cues we need to evaluate these decisions are more and more confusing, and deliberately so. Christopher Lane's study of the drafting memos behind the *DSM* categories makes it embarrassingly clear that carelessness and group-think among psychiatrists drove the creation of new categories of mental illness. Perhaps we need a "compulsive category creation" syndrome? This might be funny if there were not real-world consequences to being placed in diagnostic categories and, as Elliott would say, real money to be made in their production. Lane's chapter makes it clear that more health is not necessarily better health. Lennard Davis's chapter on the rise in obsessive-compulsive disorder (OCD) diagnoses leads us through a crucial question we have to learn to ask: given news of a new disease or an epidemic-sized increase in a scary diagnosis, how do we know we are all talking about a disorder that has been measured in the same way over time? Many of the chapters in this book remind us again and again that the answer is probably, "We don't. Condition X has come to be named and changed over time in complex ways." Davis calls this "disease made by committee" and reminds us to keep criticizing the results of this committee work just as vigorously as any other cultural product.

And finally, some critics are opposed to understandings of health that fail to place it in relationship to power structures like the organization of work and the economy, global power, and national security. Lauren Berlant declares that she is not actually against health. But she reminds us that just trying to get by can be exhausting, and pursuing pleasure to relieve that exhaustion often improves our mental health at the expense of other aspects of health. Privileged people, she points out, have a much easier time getting relief from the exhaustion of work in ways that are more healthy overall—relaxing vacations with some hiking and sleeping in, for example. Joseph Masco reminds us that we live in a security context formed from the atomic bomb (and now the suicide bomber) in which the responsible citizen should always be vigilant against the possibility of death. The dominance of a particular way of researching health also determines what kinds of global interventions will be accepted. As Vincanne Adams explains, community health workers in Karachi might know that hand washing helps to prevent the spread of diarrhea in children, but it took a double-blind controlled study in the journals to prove it to the international medical community. As it turns out, recruiting research subjects is quite a different thing from treating problems of disease, sanitation, clean water, and childbirth complications in poor countries. It might seem that health-related research is always in the service of better health, but again, we must remember to assess exactly what kind of health is being produced, for whom, according to what definitions, and under what unquestioned assumptions.

If health is really such a complex and debatable concept, there must be alternative ways of defining it. Richard Klein recommends an epicurean alternative in which health is tied to pleasure and individual freedom. Joan Wolf's practical recommendation that mothers weigh the costs and benefits of breastfeeding versus formula-feeding and do what fits best in their lives considered as a whole also values freedom as a part of health. Infant feeding is one part of one's life plan that should not have automatic veto power over other parts. Kathleen LeBesco presents the Health at Every Size (HAES) paradigm as an alternative to views of health that are overly fixated on thinness. Some of these solutions are individual-level, aesthetic alternatives, while other possibilities might be more social or structural in focus. For example, any healthcare reform that involves a national health plan would help to supplant a personal risk responsibility frame with a risk-sharing frame for health. Sharing risks means assuming that everyone has vulnerabilities over the life span and that health problems can strike anyone, even those who try to do everything right. Such a view would regard disability not as an aberration or a personal tragedy, but as part of being human. We experience a decline in our abilities as we age even if we have not been labeled "disabled" in youth or adulthood, and of course we were all completely helpless as babies. In such a view, one would not ask how much another person is going to cost, but rather how we can equitably fund a system that ensures dignity and equal citizenship for all, keeping in mind that some people will inevitably incur more medical costs than others. We might also stop thinking of health as the absence of abnormality, especially as abnormality is defined more and more widely. Disability rights advocates have been urging us to back away from rigidly enforced boundaries between the normal and the abnormal and to look instead to what a reasonably free and dignified life would look like for everyone, regardless of their ability to measure up to norms of health. These suggestions make clear that alternative ways of thinking about health are tied to necessary shifts in our thinking about concepts like risk, normality, vulnerability, accessibility, pleasure, and equality.

Our primary goal has been to dethrone health from its position of false neutrality and to insist that it be sunk down in all the complexities of political and social life in the contemporary United States. Health has long been a complex force in culture, and we are not the first to criticize the moralizing tone behind much health discourse. But we are at a challenging new moment in history that makes these issues particularly pressing. First, the powers arrayed in the health business have never been so great. Carl Elliott and Christopher Lane explain exactly how easy it is to invent and sell a new disease. While we need profitable pharmaceutical companies, large-scale food growers and processors, and yes, even distasteful products like pesticides and weapons, these entities are so vast, well-connected, and wealthy that the average citizen has very little leverage against them.

Second, we in the United States must manage health risks on an individual level without much of a collective safety net. But even if we try our best to be healthy, it is impossible to insure ourselves against every possible contingency or vulnerability. Aging and disability will come to us all if we are lucky to live long enough. Definitions of health that are really about narrowing the definition of normal so that practically everyone is diagnosable with some disorder mean that there are more groundless worries and inevitable deficiencies. The push to be healthy at an individual level reinforces an untenable presumption of personal control that is deeply at odds with the realities of our lives. The expectation is that we insure our own retirement through market investments earned through work (hoping not to rely only on Social Security), get health insurance through our employers, and take personal responsibility for our own health through diet, exercise, stress reduction, and vigilance over ourselves and our children. Of course, not everyone can achieve this standard of self-care through work because not everyone works for pay. Even those who work may find that the dangers and stresses of their jobs are themselves a challenge to health, as Lauren Berlant's chapter makes clear. Cancer, accidents, Alzheimer's, and more still strike those who do everything the experts said would prevent these misfortunes. Total self-care and independence is an illusion, inflating the sense of entitlement of those who think they have achieved it, causing unbearable stress on those who can barely achieve it, and leaving only second-class citizenship for those who cannot achieve it at all.

Third, those who strive for health exist in a paralyzing balance between deep cynicism (of profiteering companies, of contamination we cannot sense but know is there, of experts we can't trust) and the duty to act on good information (by educating ourselves on the Internet, by trying to sort the real science from the junk science). Feeling obligated yet mistrustful means that one can churn about endlessly or just grab onto something. The bigger problem beyond the individual struggle to make sense of health messages is that the constant churning of duty and mistrust takes on an ideological life of its own. The resulting instability creates more opportunities for crooks, hacks, and alarmists to manipulate structural imbalances of power. All three of these forces—significantly concentrated economic power, neoliberal risk management, and a widespread duty to act without trust in information— work to support and sustain each other. They operate far away, in corporate boardrooms and in actuarial tables, but they also echo within our own heads. How can we push back against them?

Some decisions about how to push back will be very personal. How should we go about making decisions that are now characterized as health decisions, like what to eat, what medicines to ask our doctors about, what to worry about, what sort of exercise to do (if any), whether to breastfeed and for how long, and so on? Does what we actually do matter more than how we think about our health? If we take seriously the concerns assembled here, it is clear that both what we do and the ways we think must change. One sug-gestion would be to change the ways we use language (which is both doing and thinking) to characterize health problems or situations. After reading Kathleen LeBesco on fat, for example, one might avoid the phrase "healthy weight" because that phrase actually operates to bestow moral and aesthetic approval upon a slender form. A wide variety of body sizes and shapes could be at healthy weights, in other words (or at least it might not be possible to tell just by looking at someone's body size whether she is healthy or not).

Perhaps the most important way that this volume proposes to change our way of thinking about health is its insistence that we become more self-aware about our moral impulses even if we doubt that it is possible (and maybe not even desirable) to distinguish them from more objective conclusions. What would this self-awareness look like, though, when we have acknowledged how general our mistrust of information is? There are still concrete ways to see the morality of health. We might ask, for example, if undertaking a certain health practice imparts a sense of belonging to a community. Does it contribute to an ability to sort other people based on their degrees of similarity to oneself? Are the results of this sorting hierarchically arranged, so that some people seem pitiful, oblivious, or contemptible while others are praiseworthy or even enviable? If the answer to any of these questions is yes, then we should acknowledge that health status occupies the same type of place in many people's self-concepts as do many other deeply meaningful identifications, like religion, ethnic background, nationality, and other affinities.

These affinities are extremely valuable and make our lives meaningful. There is nothing wrong with them per se. Some of them may be so deeply embedded in our senses of ourselves that it is nearly impossible to stand back from them and consider them as socially constructed, contingent, or open to change. (It is still good to give it a try.) The unusual thing about health at this moment in time, however, is that it is simultaneously becoming more and more available as a source of self-concept and achievement at the same time as it is more and more propped up by powerful economic and research interests, forceful and overblown rhetoric, public panic and misinformation, and a very solid and shiny veneer of scientific validity. These features mean that health seems to be much more neutral than it is, allowing us to pretend that we are not taking on a moral view when we aim for health. We should politicize the phrase "health status" by emphasizing the "status" part: health and the appearance of health confer status on some and take it away from others.

Another practical feature of this self-awareness should be some healthy suspicion of media presentations of health issues. As Carl Elliott's chapter on pharmaceutical public relations shows, the specific focus of our desire for health can be produced and manipulated. Once we know the level of health consciousness and status anxiety that pervades our society, it is only reasonable to expect that anyone who needs to sell newspapers, books, or advertising time, get a grant, or attract more viewers to his blog will be very likely to emphasize the dramatic and threatening aspects of any health story. We should try to maintain this suspicion, especially when the story affirms something we already believe or comes from a trusted source. Many people who are big believers in health morality already practice heightened suspicion of some media sources, usually the mainstream media or anything too connected to big corporations or the government. But this skepticism is often so highly partisan that alternative sources that are in accord with their views get little scrutiny.

We also need reforms that will make it easier for us as democratic citizens to hold powerful people accountable and to be more reflective about how we understand our health. Most of these reforms will be about money—what to do about the fact that we need large investments in health research but that those same large sums of money will produce incentives of their own, some of which will be quite damaging. The targets should be the usual bugbears in the pharmaceutical industry, but should also include those closer to home: university grant recipients, granting agencies, journal editors and reviewers, journalists and their editors, and media decision-makers. The goal of reforms should be to create greater transparency, increase the wisdom of regulation, and insert more points of independent review into the process of generating scientific truths about health.

So much of this book has been dedicated to inveighing against moralism that it is worth reflecting on the benefits of moral pressure. Conservatives, after all, have long argued that societies should enforce morality because it is the key to basic political order and happiness. Liberals often respond that we should not legislate morality. What liberals more often mean is that certain moral codes, like religious rules against homosexuality, should not be put in the law; they do not mean that deception in the form of fraud should be legal. If this is the case, then we are right back to debating exactly what moral rules should be generalized in the law and in what contexts. One impulse might be to say that health is about empirical facts and that is why it should not be moralized. It would be easy to insist, "Stop your moralizing! Just read what the scientific experts say!" But we are not taking the easy way out here. It is not our argument that science stands opposed to morality and that we should simply seek scientific objectivity and jettison morality. We are in the much tougher position of understanding *both* scientific knowledge and morality as deeply contingent and constructed but also as indispensable in the contemporary world.

We do not think expert knowledge is beyond politics and morality, nor do we wish it were. Moral intuitions may be hardwired into our brains; at the very least, it is clear that moral feelings cannot be bound to some areas of life and kept out of others. Very deep and lifelong attachments to ideas about right and wrong, whatever their source, are usually a help to organizing societies. (Of course, disagreement about these things is also the source of great violence and suffering.) But psychologists have learned a lot about how people use stereotypes and biases to keep their views from being threatened by new information or by people from outside their trusted social groups. These more petty features of our minds—inwardness, obstinacy, the tendency to ignore information that might unsettle our views—also make up the moral instinct and more crucially, enforce its boundaries. There are things we can do to combat the worst of these impulses. That is why we invented antidiscrimination law, double-blind studies, anonymous peer review of academic work, and secret ballot elections. None of these tools are perfect. The struggle to contain the worst features of moralism and squeeze as much social order from it as we can is ongoing, and exactly what that means ought to be up to democratic debate, even as we hem it in with antidemocratic measures like minority rights and civil liberties.

At the beginning of this book, we cautioned that we are not against medical treatment, nor do we mean to celebrate sickness just to be contrary. Rather, we are convinced that challenging health—being against health in certain ways—will actually promote better conversations in pivotal moments like those that occur in the doctor's office. What might be different about such an encounter after someone has read this book? Suppose a patient is discussing test results that show borderline abnormality in bone density, cholesterol, or blood pressure. The usual presumption would be that the test has indeed detected some objective feature of the patient's body that we can label, just as if he had a burn or a broken bone. An abnormal result might cause anxiety, even if the person continued to feel perfectly fine. Perhaps there would be more tests, some medication, and a label like "osteopenia" or "pre-diabetic." Certainly strong skepticism shared between the doctor and the patient would be helpful in thinking through the matter. What did the test actually measure? How was it developed and defined, and how did it change over time? Would the treatment regimen require giving up something pleasurable or convenient, and if so, what does the full balance of pros and cons look like? Bringing these questions into the discussion would mean first, that the measure of health (the test) had been denaturalized and made into an object of critical inquiry, and second, that alternative conceptions of health and the good life had come in to compete. In another scenario, a doctor and patient might discuss a troubling issue like the risk of developing cancer in terms that incorporate the contingency of fate, the burdens of trying to single-handedly prevent this fate, and the full range of emotions involved. These conversational threads would lessen the neoliberal sense of personal obligation to combat health risk as well as avoid making health into the new morality.

About the Contributors

VINCANNE ADAMS is Professor of Medical Anthropology at the University of California, San Francisco. She is the author, most recently, of *Doctors for Democracy: Health Professionals in the Nepal Revolution*, and editor, with Stacy L. Pigg, of *Sex and Development: Science, Sexuality, and Morality in Global Perspective*.

LAUREN BERLANT is the George M. Pullman Professor of English at the University of Chicago. Her most recent book is *The Female Complaint: The Unfinished Business of Sentimentality in American Culture*.

LENNARD J. DAVIS is Distinguished Professor of Liberal Arts and Sciences in the Departments of English, Disability and Human Development, and Medical Education at the University of Illinois at Chicago. He is the author most recently of *Obsession: A History* and *Go Ask Your Father: One Man's Obsession to Find Himself, His Origins, and the Meaning of Life through Genetic Testing*.

CARL ELLIOTT is Professor in the Center for Bioethics and the departments of Pediatrics and Philosophy at the University of Minnesota. He is the author of *Better than Well: American Medicine Meets the American Dream*.

S. LOCHLANN JAIN is Assistant Professor of Anthropology at Stanford University. She is the author of the recent *Injury: The Politics of Product Design and Safety Law in the United States*.

EUNJUNG KIM is Assistant Professor in the Gender and Women's Studies department and the Rehabilitation Psychology and Special Education department at the University of Wisconsin, Madison. Her essays have appeared in *Wagadu: Journal of Transnational Women's and Gender Studies* and *Canadian Journal of Film Studies*.

ANNA KIRKLAND is Associate Professor of Women's Studies and Political Science at the University of Michigan. She is the author of the recent *Fat Rights: Dilemmas of Difference and Personhood.*

RICHARD KLEIN is Professor of French Literature at Cornell University. He is the author of *Cigarettes Are Sublime* and the recent *Jewelry Talks: A Novel Thesis.*

CHRISTOPHER LANE is the Pearce Miller Research Professor of Literature in the English department at Northwestern University. He is the author of the recent *Shyness: How Normal Behavior Became a Sickness* and of the forthcoming study *The Age of Doubt: Tracing the Roots of Our Religious Uncertainty.*

KATHLEEN LEBESCO is Professor of Communication Arts at Manhattan Marymount College. She is the author of *Revolting Bodies? The Struggle to Redefine Fat Identity,* and editor, with Peter Naccarato, of the recent *Edible Ideologies: Representing Food and Meaning.*

JOSEPH MASCO is Associate Professor of Anthropology and of Social Sciences at the University of Chicago. He is the author of the recent *The Nuclear Borderlands: The Manhattan Project in Post–Cold War New Mexico.*

JONATHAN M. METZL is Associate Professor in the Women's Studies Department and the Department of Psychiatry at the University of Michigan, where he also directs the Program in Culture, Health, and Medicine. He is the author of *Prozac on the Couch: Prescribing Gender in the Era of Wonder Drugs* and *Protest Psychosis: How Schizophrenia Became a Black Disease.*

DOROTHY ROBERTS is Kirkland & Ellis Professor of Law and Professor in the departments of African American Studies and Sociology at Northwestern University. She is the author of *Shattered Bonds: The Color of Child Welfare* and *Killing the Black Body: Race, Reproduction, and the Meaning of Liberty.*

TOBIN SIEBERS is V. L. Parrington Collegiate Professor of Literary and Cultural Criticism in the Department of English Language and Literature at the University of Michigan. He is the author of *Disability Theory* and the recent *Disability Aesthetics.*

JOAN B. WOLF is Assistant Professor of Women's and Gender Studies at Texas A&M University. She is the author of *Harnessing the Holocaust: The Politics of Memory in France* and the forthcoming *Is Breast Really Best? Risk, Total Motherhood, and Breastfeeding in America.*

Index

Vietnam War, 107
Village Voice, 190
Vioxx (pharmaceutical), 99
Volkswagen, 93–94
Vulnerability, 29

Wall Street Journal, 4
Wal-Mart Stores, Inc., 10n6
Weber Shandwick, 102
Weight loss, 2, 16, 78–79, 81
Welch, H. Gilbert, 6
Well-being, 27
Wetzler, Scott, 115
Whitmarsh, Ian, 47
Widiger, Thomas, 115
Williams, Patricia, 186
Wine, 21
Witchcraft, 43
Women, 84, 86, 90; Asian American, 161; eating and mobility patterns of, 38n12; and fatness, 75; and genetic selection, 67; and pregnancy, 62, 83

Work, 27–28, 32, 34–35
Worker(s), 33–34, 36
Working class, 32, 75; families, 34; and breastfeeding, 89
World Alzheimer's Congress, 97–98
World Health Organization (WHO), 41, 46–47, 50, 53, 121
World Neighbors, 50
World War II, 9, 106
Wright, Jan, 76
Wrongful birth, 184, 186, 193n10
Wrongful life, 186–188, 193n10
Wyeth, 96, 99

Xigris (pharmaceutical), 101–102

Yale-Brown Obsessive Compulsive Scale (Y-BOCS), 125

Zaloom, Caitlyn, 176
Zola, Irving, 5
Zoloft (pharmaceutical), 96, 99–100